CHAIR YOGA

FOR WEIGHT LOSS

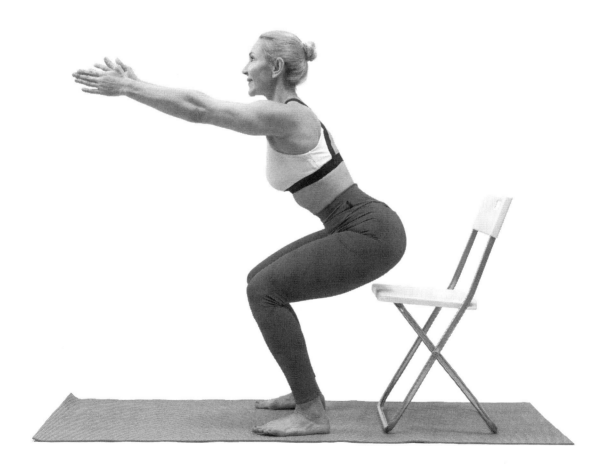

SheerFitness**Vibes**

TABLE OF CONTENTS

DISCLAIMER

The information provided in this book is intended for general informational purposes only. The author and publisher of this book are not licensed medical professionals, and the content within this book should not be considered a substitute for professional medical advice, diagnosis, or treatment. Always seek the advice of your physician or other qualified health provider with any questions you may have regarding a medical condition.

The exercises, techniques, and advice presented in this book are meant to be a general guide for chair yoga and should be performed with caution and under the guidance of a qualified instructor or healthcare provider. Individuals with pre-existing medical conditions, injuries, or physical limitations should consult with their healthcare professionals before attempting any exercises or practices outlined in this book.

The author and publisher of this book do not assume any responsibility or liability for any injury, loss, or damage that may result from the use of the information contained in this book. The reader takes full responsibility for their health and well-being and should use their best judgment when following the instructions and recommendations provided in this book.

It is important to remember that individual results may vary, and the effectiveness of chair yoga exercises may depend on various factors, including an individual's physical condition and consistency in practice.

By reading this book, you acknowledge and agree to the terms of this disclaimer. You understand that the author and publisher shall not be held responsible for any consequences arising from your use of the information contained herein.

If you do not agree with the terms of this disclaimer, please do not use the information provided in this book.

❝

"Caring for your body, mind, and spirit is your greatest and grandest responsibility. It's about listening to the needs of your soul and then honoring them."
— *Kristi Ling*

❞

INTRODUCTION

Welcome to "Chair Yoga for Weight Loss"!
By picking up this book, you're choosing a healthier and more active lifestyle. Good for you! This guide introduces you to Chair Yoga with easy tips and physical activities. The exercises provided here are separated into three different categories, aiming for relaxation, tonification and fast-fat burning, so you can pick up those that are more suited for your goals:

- **Chair Yoga Exercises:** Delve into the foundational yoga poses focusing on breathing, meditation, relaxation, and stretching. This chapter sets the stage for the rest of your journey.

- **Muscle Toning Exercises:** Here, you'll find exercises tailored to enhance muscle tonicity and strength. These are essential for building a strong and resilient body.

- **Cardio Exercises:** This chapter is all about getting your heart rate up and promoting fat burning. It's the key to weight loss and improving cardiovascular health.

Once you're familiar with the individual exercises, it's time to put them together to create your daily routine. The last two chapters are about:

- **Flows and Routines:** Here, you'll find how to combine exercises into 5-10 minute sessions. You can easily make them a daily habit. And if you'd like, you can mix them up to suit your liking!

- **28-Day Challenge:** Ready for a transformative journey? This chapter offers a detailed 28-day workout plan aimed at promoting weight loss. Each day presents one or more routines to perform, ensuring variety and comprehensive training.

Whether you follow our structured plan or create your own routines, this book is designed to be flexible and cater to your needs. Dive in, explore, and most importantly, enjoy the journey to a healthier you!

ACCESS THE VIDEO TUTORIALS

In this book, you'll notice small square patterns, known as QR codes, next to all the exercises. Think of these as magic portals to helpful videos! A QR code is like a barcode, but instead of being read at the store, you can read it with your smartphone or tablet.

To use it, simply open the camera app on your device, point it at the QR code, and a link will appear. Tap on this link, and you'll be taken directly to an instructional video that shows you how to perform the exercise.

If you have trouble using the QR code or prefer not to, don't worry! You can go to our website **www.sheerfitnessvibes.com** and access our video tutorials from there. Please note that the chair yoga section is private and requires a special code for access. But don't fret! As a purchaser of this book, you have lifetime free access. Simply turn to page 108 and follow the provided instructions.

We've included these options to make it easier for you to visualize and understand each exercise, whether you're using the QR code or the website directly.

Even if you've never used a QR code before, give it a try! It's a simple way to enhance your learning experience and ensure you're doing each exercise correctly.

Now, are you ready to dive into some activities? Let's get started!

1.

Open the camera on your smartphone and point it at the QR code for the exercise you wish to access.

2.

When you aim your camera at the QR code, a button should appear on your screen. If nothing happens, try tapping the area on your phone's screen displaying the QR code. Click the button when it appears.

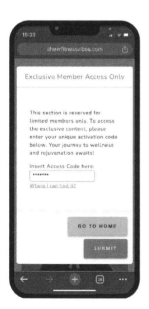

3.

You will be redirected to the video tutorial linked to the QR code. If you're using the device for the first time, you'll be asked to enter the code found on page 108. Don't fret; you'll only need to enter this code once for each device you use.

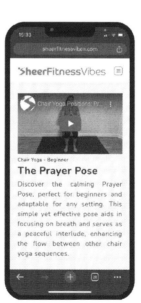

4.

Once you've entered the code, you'll have lifetime access to our video tutorials. If you encounter any issues, feel free to contact us at the following email address:

support@sheerfitnessvibes.com

MAKE THE MOST OUT OF CHAIR YOGA

PREPARATION TIPS

While chair yoga is a low-intensity practice, some preparation is essential. Ensure you haven't eaten for at least 2 hours prior to your session, and avoid drinking excessively to prevent feeling heavy during certain poses.

Before you begin, take a moment to center yourself. Set aside the events of your day, close your eyes, and breathe deeply and slowly. Let your shoulders relax and immerse yourself in the stillness. In our bustling lives, moments of true silence and introspection are rare. Seize this opportunity to create a mental sanctuary, preparing for the yoga journey ahead.

Remember, the essence of yoga isn't about the number of poses you do or the complexity of the session. It's about the tranquility of your mind and its readiness to engage with the practice. If you ever find yourself pressed for time, prioritize achieving a calm and receptive mindset before starting. Everything else can take a backseat.

1 WAIT 2 HOURS AFTER EATING

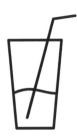

2 DON'T DRINK MUCH

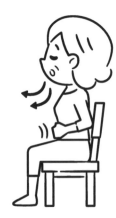

3 BREATHE DEEPLY AND SLOWLY

PICK THE RIGHT CLOTHES

While I'm not suggesting a complete wardrobe overhaul, it's essential to select attire that best supports your yoga practice from what you already own.

Comfort should be your primary consideration when dressing for yoga. Fashion trends or aesthetic appeal should take a backseat. Opt for clothing made from cotton or other natural fibers to minimize excessive sweating and potential discomfort.

Many practitioners favor leggings due to their flexibility and breathability, especially when made from quality cotton. Others choose soft sweatpants that taper at the ankles. Both are excellent choices. Similarly, for tops, go for breathable t-shirts or sweaters that offer comfort without being overly tight.

Historically, yoga was practiced barefoot, but modern adaptations welcome the use of socks for hygiene and comfort. While there are socks specifically designed for yoga, any cotton variant will suffice.

This book emphasizes chair yoga at home, where you can regulate the temperature. Nonetheless, keep a long-sleeved shirt nearby to stay warm during meditation sessions.

In terms of color, neutral shades like black, beige, gray, and white are recommended. They foster a meditative mindset and exude calmness. For those with long hair, consider tying it back or using a headband to prevent distractions. Lastly, always have a towel—preferably made of natural fibers and in soft colors—on hand to dab away sweat.

PICK THE RIGHT CHAIR

Choosing the right chair for chair yoga is paramount. The chair serves as your foundation, ensuring stability, safety, and proper alignment during exercises. Here's what to consider when selecting your chair:

- **Sturdiness:** Opt for a robust and stable chair. Chairs with wheels can move unexpectedly and should be avoided to minimize the risk of injury.

- **Width and Depth:** Your chair should be wide and deep enough for comfort, but not so expansive that your feet can't rest flat on the ground.

- **Back Support:** A straight-backed chair is ideal, offering support for various poses and promoting proper posture.

- **Cushioning:** Chairs with minimal or no cushioning are preferable. Overly soft seats can challenge your balance during certain poses.

- **Height:** Ensure that when seated, your feet touch the floor and your knees align with your hips or are slightly lower. If the chair is too tall, consider using blocks or books to support your feet.

- **Material:** Choose a chair with a non-slippery material, especially for the seat, to prevent sliding during poses.

- **No Wheels:** As emphasized, avoid chairs with wheels as they can be hazardous due to unexpected movement.

The right chair ensures you can focus on your poses and breathing, rather than worrying about wobbling or discomfort. Remember, in chair yoga, your chair isn't just a prop—it's an integral part of your journey to wellness.

CHAIR YOGA POSITIONS

PRAYER POSE

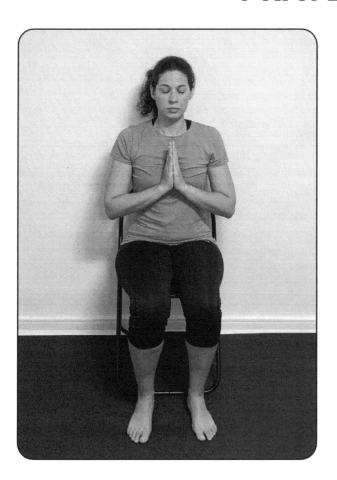

INSTRUCTIONS

1. Sit comfortably on a chair, ensuring your spine is aligned and your feet are firmly on the ground.

2. As you take a deep breath in, clasp your hands together in a prayer position and position them before your chest.

3. Make sure your elbows are relaxed and not pressed against your body. It's essential to keep your fingers, wrists, and shoulders free from tension.

4. (Optional) If you're comfortable, gently close your eyes and focus on your breathing, noticing the rhythmic movement of your body with each inhalation and exhalation.

5. Embrace any thoughts that arise, allowing them to come and go without judgment. As you center your attention on your breathing, you'll find these thoughts diminishing.

6. To conclude, slowly open your eyes, release your hands, and proceed with your next activity or pose.

✗ MISTAKES TO AVOID

- **Duration:** If you have a history of wrist or arm issues, be cautious about the duration you maintain this pose.

The Prayer Pose is ideal for beginners as it doesn't necessitate any prior preparation. Its versatility allows it to be practiced in a myriad of settings, whether you're at home, in a waiting room, or even traveling. Not only does it offer an opportunity to recenter and reconnect with one's breathing, bringing a moment of tranquility, but it also acts as a seamless transition between other chair yoga movements, providing a brief respite and focus.

SHOULDER CIRCLES

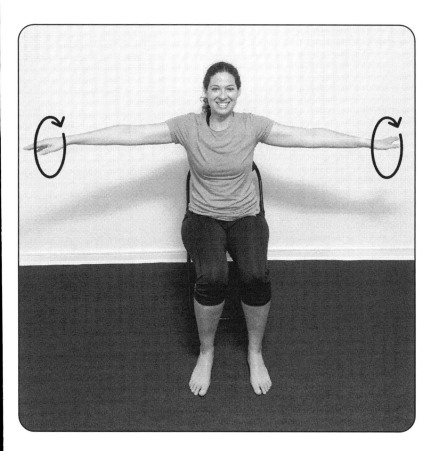

✗ MISTAKES TO AVOID

- **Rapid Movements:** Ensure the circles are slow and controlled to avoid straining the shoulders.

- **Incomplete Circles:** Make sure to utilize the full range of motion for the shoulder joint.

- **Tensing the Neck:** Keep the neck relaxed throughout the exercise to avoid unnecessary strain.

- **Improper Breathing:** Breathing should be synchronized with the movement. Avoid holding your breath or breathing too rapidly.

The Shoulder Circles exercise is a dynamic movement aimed at increasing flexibility and relieving tension in the shoulder joints. By methodically rotating the shoulders in synchronized circles, practitioners can combat the rigidity often stemming from prolonged sitting or repetitive tasks. This exercise not only fosters improved range of motion but also aids in strengthening the surrounding musculature, making it an essential practice for maintaining shoulder health and promoting overall upper body well-being.

INSTRUCTIONS

1. Begin by sitting upright on a chair, ensuring your spine is tall and aligned.

2. Extend your arms straight out to your sides, keeping them level with your shoulders.

3. With your arms extended, start making small circular movements focused on the shoulder joint. Ensure the rotation is subtle and your arms remain mostly at shoulder level.

4. Throughout the exercise, maintain steady and constant breathing through your nostrils.

5. Ensure the movement is smooth and controlled, emphasizing the rotation in the shoulder while keeping the arms straight. Remember to breathe consistently and calmly as you perform the rotations.

SIDE TWIST

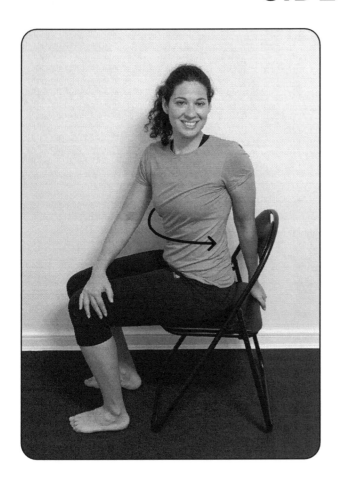

INSTRUCTIONS

1. Begin by sitting on a chair, ensuring your back is straight and your feet are flat on the ground.

2. As you inhale, lengthen your spine, imagining you are creating space between the vertebrae. Keep your shoulders rolled back and relaxed.

3. Exhale and gently twist your torso towards the left. Place your left hand on the back of the chair and your right hand outside your left thigh. Deepen the twist with each exhale, ensuring your shoulders remain away from your ears.

4. Turn your head to the left, gazing over your left shoulder. Hold the position for a few breaths.

5. Inhale and release, returning to the starting position.

6. Follow the same steps, twisting towards the right side.

X MISTAKES TO AVOID

- **Over-Twisting:** Avoid twisting too aggressively, which can strain the spine.

- **Holding Breath:** Maintain consistent breathing throughout the pose.

- **Jerky Movements:** Move smoothly and avoid any sudden jerks.

The Side Twist is a rejuvenating seated movement designed to enhance spinal flexibility and alleviate tension in the torso. By methodically twisting the upper body, practitioners can counteract the stiffness often associated with prolonged desk work or sedentary lifestyles. This pose not only promotes better posture but also aids in detoxifying the body, making it a valuable addition to any chair yoga routine or daily stretching regimen.

FOLD POSE

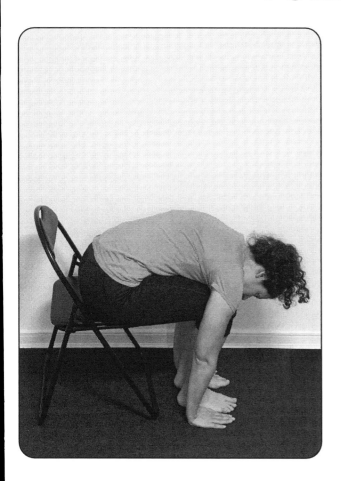

INSTRUCTIONS

1. Begin by sitting comfortably on a chair, ensuring your spine is extended and your breathing is relaxed.

2. As you inhale, lengthen your torso upwards.

3. On your exhale, gently bend forward from your hips, bringing your arms down towards your feet.

4. Allow your torso to rest on your thighs, positioning your chin close to your knees. Direct your gaze downward towards your feet.

5. As you take deep breaths, gently move your torso towards your thighs. Try to extend your shoulders to place your palms on the floor, but remember, it's okay if you can't get your entire palm down. Everyone's range of movement is different, so work within yours and make sure not to strain your back. It's all about what feels right for you.

6. Stay in this position for a couple of breaths, deepening the stretch with each exhale.

7. To come out of the pose, inhale and look up first. Then, raise your arms upwards and return to the seated position.

✗ MISTAKES TO AVOID

- **Overstretching:** Avoid pushing too hard or trying to go deeper than your body allows. Listen to your body and move within a comfortable range.

- **Holding Breath:** Ensure you breathe consistently throughout the pose.

- **Not using Props:** Consider placing a cushion on your thighs for added support if breathing is challenging.

- **Feet Placement:** Ensure your feet remain flat on the ground for stability.

The Fold Pose is a therapeutic exercise tailored for those seeking the benefits of traditional forward folds without the strain. Performed from a seated position, this pose emphasizes a gentle forward bend, targeting the upper body and spine. It's an ideal stretch for individuals who spend extended hours seated, offering relief from tension and promoting spinal flexibility. With its adaptability, including the use of props, it caters to various physical conditions, making it a versatile addition to any chair yoga routine or relaxation regimen.

LOW LUNGE

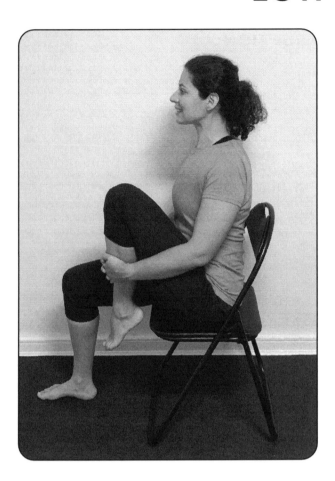

INSTRUCTIONS

1. Sit comfortably on a chair. Ensure your spine is extended, and your feet are firmly placed on the floor. Lengthen your spine and relax your shoulders.

2. Inhale and lift your left leg, bending the knee. Use your hands to support the leg.

3. As you exhale, press the thigh closer to your chest, flexing the left ankle. Point your toes downward and maintain a straight back, bringing the knee as close to your chest as possible.

4. Hold the position for a few breaths, feeling the stretch in the hips, pelvic floor muscles, lower back, and core muscles.

5. Exhale, release the left leg, and place both feet on the floor. Adjust your position if necessary, then repeat the steps with the right leg.

✗ MISTAKES TO AVOID

- **Overstretching:** Avoid pressing the thigh too aggressively towards the chest, which can strain the hip flexors.

- **Misalignment:** Ensure your back remains straight throughout the pose. Avoid rounding or arching excessively.

- **Holding Breath:** Breathe consistently throughout the pose.

- **Lack of Support:** If lifting the leg is challenging, consider using props or modifications to support the leg.

The Low Lunge is a gentle seated stretch designed to open the hip flexors and engage the core muscles. By methodically lifting and pressing the leg towards the chest, practitioners can counteract the stiffness often associated with prolonged sitting. This pose not only promotes better hip mobility but also aids in strengthening the core, making it a valuable addition to any chair yoga routine or daily stretching regimen.

COBRA

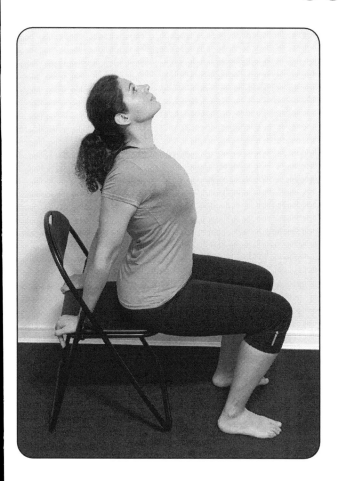

INSTRUCTIONS

1. Sit at the front edge of your chair, ensuring your feet are flat on the ground and hip-distance apart. Lengthen your spine, ensuring your back is straight.

2. Place your hands on the back of the chair, holding it firmly.

3. As you inhale, lift your chest towards the ceiling, arching your back slightly. Allow your gaze to move upwards, feeling an opening in the chest.

4. Maintain this arched position, feeling the stretch in your upper back and chest. Ensure your neck remains relaxed and avoid straining it.

5. Exhale and return to the starting position.

✗ MISTAKES TO AVOID

- **Over-Arching:** Avoid excessive arching of the back, which can strain the spine and neck.

- **Straining the Neck:** Ensure your neck remains relaxed and avoid throwing your head back too far.

- **Gripping Too Tightly:** While holding the chair, avoid gripping too tightly, which can create tension in the arms and shoulders.

The Chair Cobra Pose is a gentle seated backbend designed to open the chest and stretch the upper back. By methodically arching the spine while seated, practitioners can counteract the stiffness often associated with prolonged desk work or sedentary lifestyles. This pose not only promotes better posture but also aids in revitalizing the spine, making it a valuable addition to any chair yoga routine or daily stretching regimen.

ONE-LEGGED SEATED FORWARD BEND

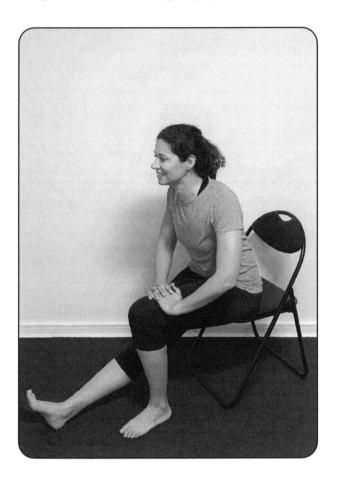

INSTRUCTIONS

1. Sit comfortably on a chair, ensuring your spine is straight and your feet are flat on the ground, hip-distance apart.

2. Slowly extend your right leg straight out in front of you, keeping the heel resting on the ground and toes pointing upwards.

3. As you inhale, lengthen your spine, lifting your chest upwards.

4. As you exhale, place your hands on your left thigh, hinge at the hips and bend forward. Aim to bring your chest towards your thigh.

5. Hold this position for several breaths, feeling the stretch in the back of the extended leg.

6. Inhale and slowly come back to an upright position. Switch legs and repeat the process.

The One-Legged Seated Forward Bend in Chair Yoga offers a gentle yet effective way to stretch the hamstrings and calves. By focusing on one leg at a time, practitioners can address imbalances and ensure a thorough stretch. This pose is particularly beneficial for those who spend long hours sitting, as it helps counteract tightness in the legs and promotes better circulation. Regular practice can lead to improved flexibility and reduced tension in the lower body.

✗ MISTAKES TO AVOID

- **Rounding the Back:** Ensure you hinge from the hips and keep your spine long as you bend forward.

- **Overstretching:** Listen to your body and only bend forward to a point that feels comfortable. Avoid pushing too hard.

- **Lifting the Extended Leg's Heel:** Ensure the heel of the extended leg remains grounded throughout the pose.

- **Holding Breath:** Breathe consistently throughout the pose, coordinating each movement with your breath.

PIGEON STRETCH

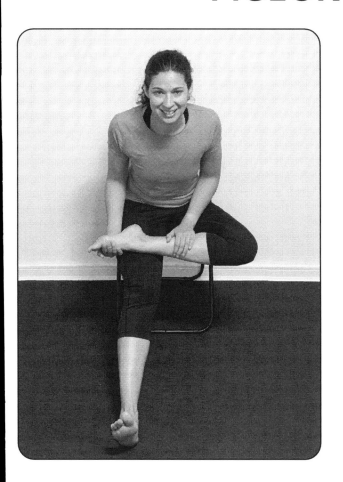

INSTRUCTIONS

1. Sit comfortably on a chair, ensuring your spine is straight and your feet are flat on the ground.

2. Lift your right leg, holding it gently with your hands. Place it over your left thigh.

3. Slowly extend your left leg straight out in front of you, keeping the heel resting on the ground and toes pointing upwards.

4. As you inhale, lengthen your torso upwards.

5. On your exhale, gently bend forward from your hips. You will feel the hip joint and the knee flexing.

6. After a few breaths, go back to your original position and repeat the process with your left leg.

X MISTAKES TO AVOID

- **Overstretching:** Ensure you don't force your leg into a position that feels uncomfortable or painful.

- **Incorrect Foot Placement:** Make sure you always keep one heel resting on the ground.

- **Rushing the Pose:** Take your time to get into the pose and ensure you're comfortable before proceeding.

The Chair Pigeon Pose is a seated variation of the traditional Pigeon Pose, tailored for those who might find the floor version challenging. By elevating the practice to a chair, it offers a more accessible way to open the hips and stretch the lower body. This pose is particularly beneficial for those who spend extended periods sitting, as it helps counteract stiffness and promotes better circulation in the legs.

HANDS UP

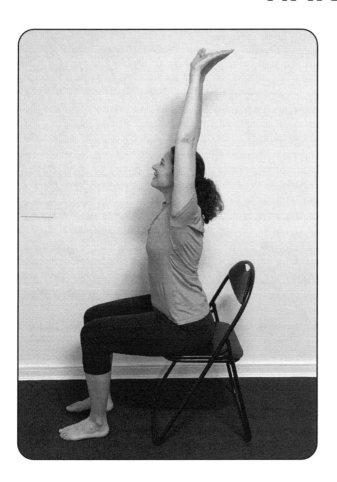

INSTRUCTIONS

1. Sit comfortably on a chair, ensuring your spine is straight and your feet are flat on the ground.

2. As you inhale, lift your arms above your head, opening the chest and stretching the shoulders and arms completely.

3. Exhale once you're in position and maintain the pose for 1-2 breaths.

4. Exhale and gently lower your arms back to the starting position.

✗ MISTAKES TO AVOID

- **Overstretching:** Avoid raising your arms too forcefully or beyond a comfortable range.

- **Holding Breath:** Ensure you breathe consistently throughout the pose. Holding your breath can lead to tension.

- **Rapid Movements:** Move your arms in a controlled and deliberate manner, avoiding any jerky motions.

The Hands Up Pose focuses on stretching the upper body, particularly the arms and shoulders. By raising the arms above the head, practitioners can experience a gentle opening of the chest and improved circulation. This pose is especially beneficial for those who spend extended periods sitting, as it helps counteract stiffness and promotes better upper body flexibility.

HIGH LUNGE

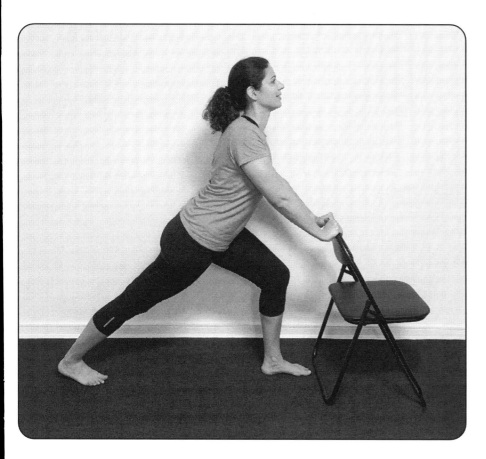

High Lunge Chair Variation is a beginner-level standing yoga pose. It targets the hamstrings, hips, and quadriceps, strengthening the legs and enhancing balance and core stability. As with any yoga pose, ensure proper alignment and work within your flexibility and strength limits.

INSTRUCTIONS

1. Begin by standing upright in front of your chair.

2. Take a step back with your right foot, placing it flat on the ground. Your left foot remains forward, with the knee bent. Hold onto the seat for support.

3. Ensure that your hips are squared and facing forward.

4. Maintain this position for a few deep breaths, feeling the stretch in the front of your right hip and the engagement of your left thigh.

5. Step your right foot forward to return to the starting position. Repeat on the opposite side.

✗ MISTAKES TO AVOID

- **Overextending the Knee:** Ensure your front knee is directly above the ankle, not extending past the toes.

- **Misaligned Hips:** Keep your hips squared and facing forward. Avoid letting one hip dip or rise higher than the other.

- **Holding Breath:** Breathe consistently throughout the pose to maintain balance and relaxation.

WARRIOR POSE

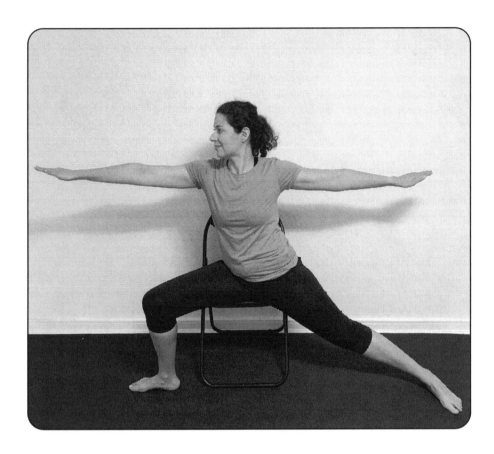

This Warrior Pose is a modified version, adapted for those who may need additional support or are looking for a less intense variation. This pose helps in strengthening the legs, opening the hips, and stretching the arms and upper body. It also aids in improving balance and concentration.

INSTRUCTIONS

1. Begin by sitting comfortably on a chair, keeping your spine straight.

2. Open your right leg to create a 90-degree angle between your legs. Bend your right knee, ensuring it aligns directly over your foot. Your foot should be parallel to your leg.

3. Shift your sitting position to the left, allowing the chair to support your right leg.

4. Extend your left leg straight out and position your left foot diagonally, creating approximately between a 45-degree and a 60-degree angle with your right foot.

5. Keep your hips facing forward and extend your arms out at shoulder height. Direct your gaze to the right.

6. Engage your abdomen and elongate your spine to maintain balance and stability in the pose.

7. Hold this position for 3-5 breaths, feeling the stretch along the inner thighs and the engagement of your arms.

8. To exit the pose, straighten your right knee, lower your arms, and bring your feet back to hip-width apart.

✗ MISTAKES TO AVOID

- **Overextending the Front Knee:** Ensure your front knee doesn't go past your ankle. This can strain the knee joint.

- **Misalignment of the Feet:** Ensure your front foot points directly forward and the back foot is angled correctly.

- **Losing Balance:** Use the chair for support, and your extended arms for balance.

HUMBLE WARRIOR POSE

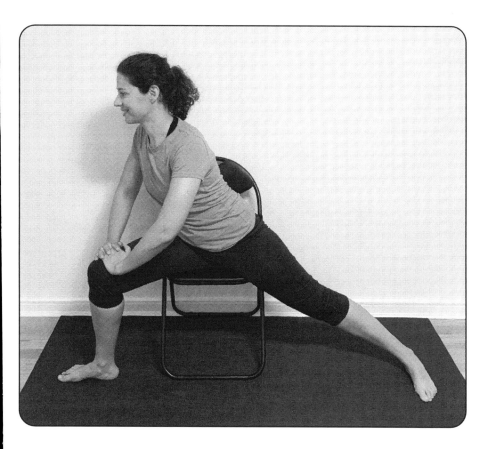

This is a beginner-level yoga pose executed in a sitting position, incorporating a forward bend. This variation of the traditional Humble Warrior Pose targets the legs, hips, arms, chest, rib cage, shoulders, spine, and core muscles, offering a comprehensive stretch and engagement for these areas.

INSTRUCTIONS

1. Begin by ensuring you're seated comfortably on a chair with your spine straight.

2. Position your feet a comfortable distance apart. Turn your front foot (the one closest to the chair) to point directly forward, and angle your back foot slightly inwards, approximately 45 degrees.

3. Bend your front knee, making sure it aligns directly over your ankle. Ensure your knee points in the same direction as your front foot.

4. Adjust your seated position slightly to accommodate more of your forward leg on the chair.

5. Place your hands on your front knee with fingers interlocked. Keep the el-bows bent and pointed to the sides.

6. Keep the chest broad and lifted, with a gentle twist and a slight forward bend. Ensure the chin is aligned with the chest and slightly tucked in. Keep the shoulders broad. Look downwards.

7. Exhale as you bend forward. Hold the position for a few breaths and release. Repeat on the opposite side.

X MISTAKES TO AVOID

- Overextending the legs or placing too much pressure on the knees.

- Slouching or not keeping the spine straight and lifted.

- Not engaging the core muscles, leading to strain on the lower back.

SUN BREATHS

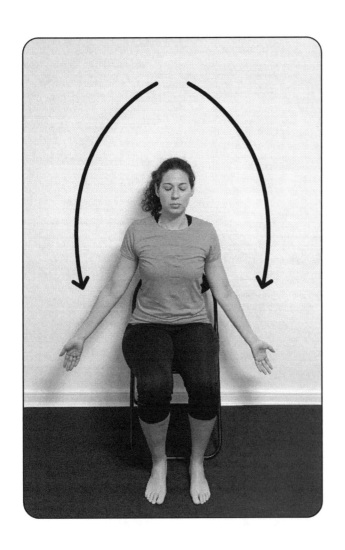 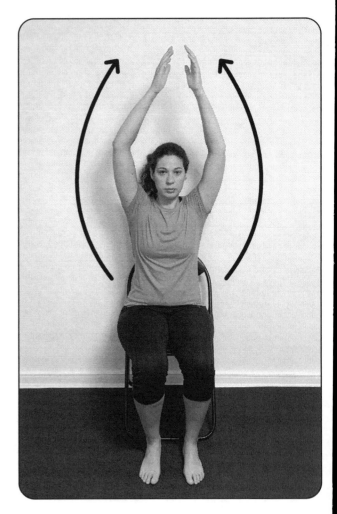

The Sun Breaths pose offers a serene way to anchor oneself while deepening the connection to one's breathing. Beyond fostering breath mindfulness, this pose provides a gentle stretch to the upper torso, encouraging improved posture. Especially beneficial for those who spend long hours seated, it serves as a relief, alleviating strain from the neck and shoulders.

INSTRUCTIONS

1. Start by positioning yourself upright on a chair, ensuring your feet are firmly planted on the floor and spaced hip-width apart. Maintain a straight spine and let your shoulders ease into a relaxed stance.

2. Initiate the exercise by drawing a deep breath in through your nostrils, allowing the inhalation to guide your movements.

3. As you breathe in, lift your arms in a sweeping motion with palms facing forward. Ensure your shoulders remain at ease as you extend your arms overhead.

4. When exhaling, release the breath through your nostrils slightly before you begin to lower your arms. Slightly rotate your palms outward as you gracefully bring your arms back down to your sides.

5. Continue this pattern several times, letting each breath and movement bring you closer to a state of calm and centeredness.

✗ MISTAKES TO AVOID

- **Holding Breath:** The pose is meant to synchronize with breathing. Holding one's breath or not coordinating the movements with inhalation and exhalation can diminish the calming effects of the pose.

- **Raising the Shoulders:** When extending the arms, there's a tendency for some to raise their shoulders, which can cause tension in the neck and upper back. It's essential to keep the shoulders relaxed and down.

NECK ROLLS

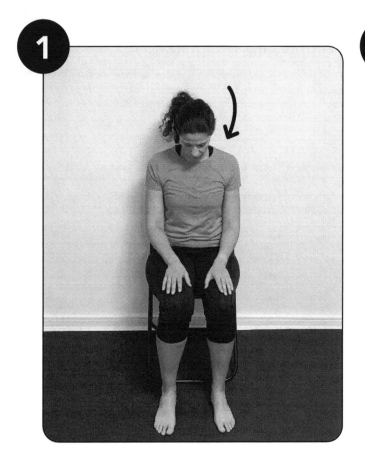

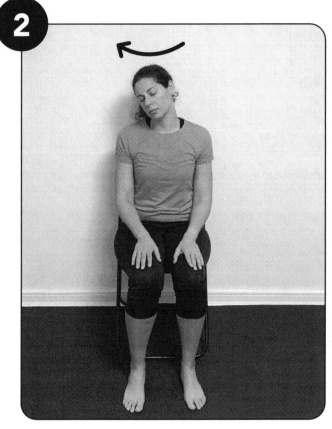

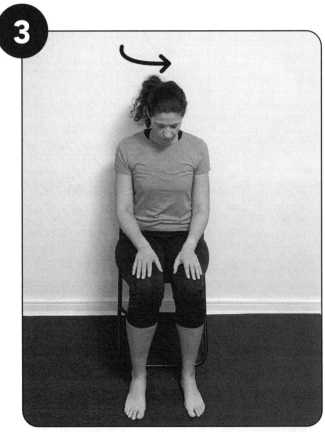

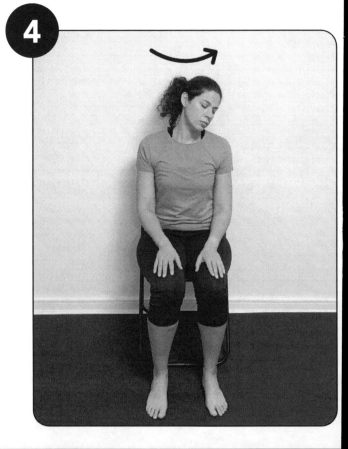

For individuals who often find themselves hunched over a computer or desk for extended periods, Seated Neck Rolls offer a remarkable solution to ease neck tension and stiffness. Embarking on this exercise with a few rotations and progressively increasing the count as familiarity and comfort grow is advisable. With consistent practice, not only does this pose enhance neck flexibility, but it also paves the way for improved posture, fostering overall spinal health.

INSTRUCTIONS

1. Inhale deeply and gently lower your chin towards your chest, feeling a subtle stretch in the back of your neck.

2. Slowly rotate your head to the right, aiming to bring your right ear closer to your right shoulder without straining.

3. Exhale and guide your chin back to your chest in a controlled motion.

4. Inhale and gently turn your head to the left, attempting to bring your left ear towards your left shoulder with ease.

   Exhale and return your chin to your chest, finalizing one full neck rotation.

✗ MISTAKES TO AVOID

- **Overstretching:** It's essential not to force the neck into any position. The rotations should be gentle, and you should never feel pain.

- **Rapid Movements:** Avoid making quick or jerky movements. The rotations should be slow and controlled.

- **Lifting the Shoulders:** Some might unconsciously lift their shoulders while rotating the neck. Ensure your shoulders remain relaxed and down throughout the exercise.

- **Holding Breath:** Breathing should be consistent and not held during the rotations.

NECK ROLLS - DOWN & UP

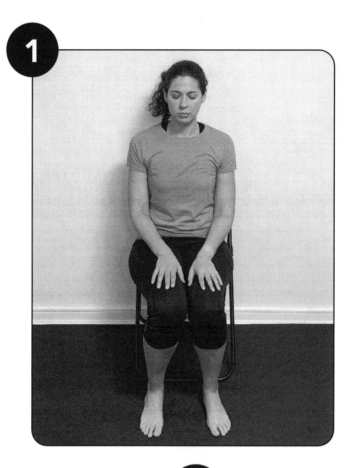

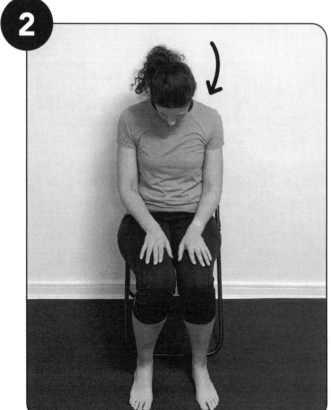

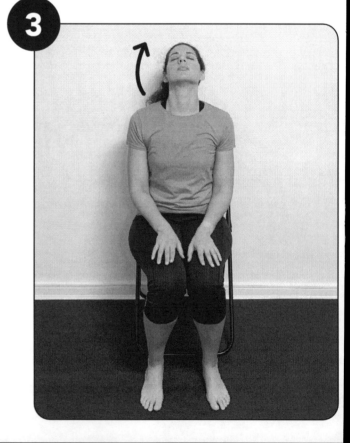

Neck Rolls Down & Up, emphasizing the up and down motion, are a simple yet effective seated exercise to alleviate neck tension. By mindfully tilting the head forward and backward, practitioners can enhance cervical flexibility, counteract stiffness, and promote a relaxed neck posture. Ideal for those seeking a quick relief from prolonged stationary positions, this exercise is a go-to for neck rejuvenation.

INSTRUCTIONS

1. Sit comfortably on a chair with your feet flat on the ground, hip-width apart. Ensure your spine is erect, shoulders are relaxed, and hands rest on your lap or knees. Begin with your head in a centered position, eyes looking straight ahead.

2. Inhale and maintain a relaxed posture. Exhale as you gently lower your chin towards your chest, feeling a light stretch along the back of your neck. Ensure you're moving only your head and not leaning your upper body forward.

3. Inhale as you slowly lift your head, tilting it backward. Allow your eyes to gaze upwards, stretching the front of your neck. Be cautious not to strain; tilt only as far back as comfortable. Exhale and return your head to the neutral position.

✗ MISTAKES TO AVOID

- **Tensing the Shoulders:** Some people unconsciously raise or tense their shoulders while doing neck rolls. The shoulders should remain relaxed and down throughout the exercise.

- **Using the Upper Body:** Leaning the upper body forward or backward instead of isolating the movement to the neck is a common mistake. The spine should remain straight, and only the neck should move.

SIDE STRETCH

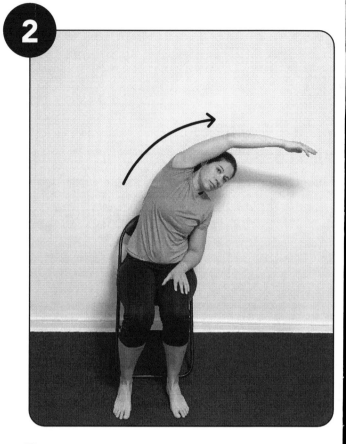

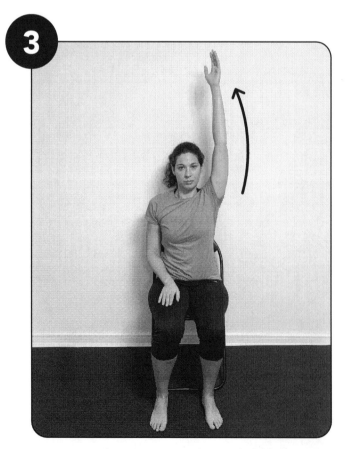

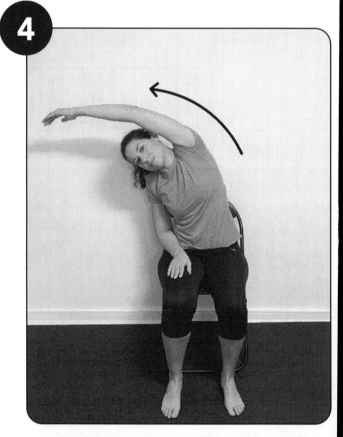

The Chair Seated Side Stretch Pose offers a gentle yet effective way to stretch and open the side body, particularly targeting the shoulders and neck. Ideal for those seeking a break from desk work or prolonged sitting, this pose provides both relaxation and rejuvenation. Using a chair as a prop ensures stability and accessibility, making it suitable for practitioners of all levels.

INSTRUCTIONS

1. Begin by sitting upright in a chair, ensuring your spine is straight, and your feet are flat on the ground. Inhale as you lift your right arm upwards.

2. Extend your right arm towards the left side while gently tilting your chest and neck to the left. Exhale and hold this position, taking a few deep breaths. Maintain your balance without leaning too far to the left. After a few seconds, slowly return to your starting position, beginning with your chest and then lowering your arm alongside your body. Place your right hand on your right thigh.

3. Now, let's perform the same movement on the left side. Inhale and lift your left arm upwards.

4. Gently tilt your chest and neck to the left while extending your left arm towards the left side. Hold this position for 2-3 seconds before gradually returning to your original position.

✗ MISTAKES TO AVOID

- **Overstretching:** Ensure you don't lean too far to one side, which can cause strain or imbalance.

- **Holding Breath:** Maintain consistent breathing throughout the pose to ensure relaxation and proper oxygen flow.

- **Rapid Movements:** Move slowly and deliberately to avoid any sudden jerks or strains.

- **Improper Hand Placement:** Ensure your non-stretching hand is resting comfortably on the chair or your lap for stability.

CAT COW

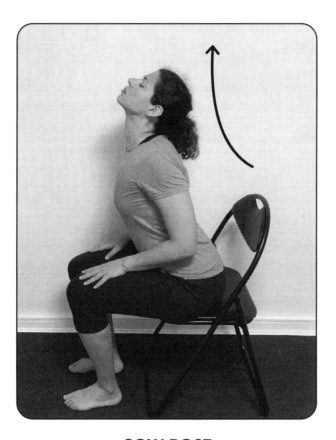

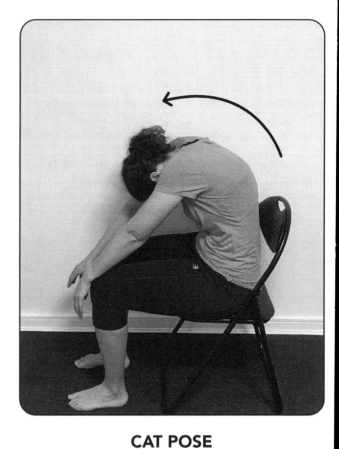

COW POSE

As you **inhale**, arch your back slightly, pushing your chest forward and lifting your chin

CAT POSE

As you **exhale**, round your spine, tucking your chin towards your chest and drawing your navel towards your spine.

The Chair Cat Cow Pose is a dynamic seated movement designed to enhance spinal flexibility and alleviate tension in the back. By methodically arching and rounding the spine, practitioners can counteract the stiffness often associated with prolonged desk work or sedentary lifestyles. This pose not only promotes better posture but also aids in revitalizing the spine, making it a valuable addition to any chair yoga routine or daily stretching regimen.

INSTRUCTIONS

1. Begin by sitting near the front of the chair seat, ensuring your feet are hip-distance apart and firmly planted under your knees. Ensure your spine is straight and your hands are placed on or near your knees.

2. As you inhale, arch your back slightly, pushing your chest forward and lifting your chin, allowing your gaze to move upwards. Your shoulder blades should move down your back.

3. As you exhale, round your spine, tucking your chin towards your chest and drawing your navel towards your spine. Feel the stretch along your back.

4. Continue to flow between these two positions, inhaling into Cow Pose and exhaling into Cat Pose, for several breath cycles.

5. After completing the desired number of repetitions, return to a neutral spine and relax.

✗ MISTAKES TO AVOID

- **Over-Arching or Over-Rounding:** Avoid excessive arching or rounding of the spine, which can cause strain.

- **Holding Breath:** Ensure you breathe consistently throughout the pose, coordinating each movement with your breath.

- **Rapid Movements:** Move in a controlled manner, ensuring each movement is smooth and deliberate.

- **Lack of Alignment:** Ensure your feet remain flat on the ground and your hands maintain their position on your knees.

ASSISTED LEG EXTENSIONS

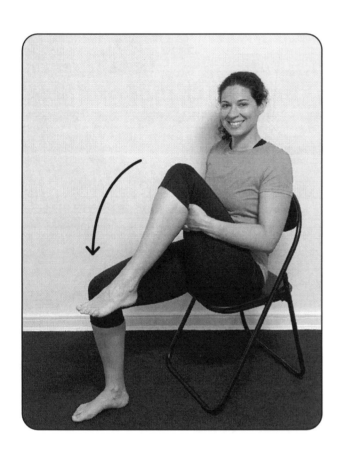
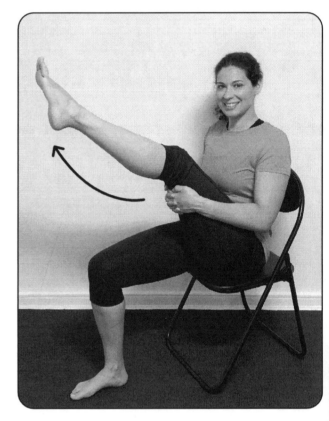

Assisted Leg Extensions in chair yoga offer a targeted way to engage and strengthen the quadriceps muscles. By methodically lifting and lowering one leg at a time, practitioners can focus on muscle engagement and control. This exercise is particularly beneficial for those looking to improve leg strength without putting strain on the joints. Regular practice can lead to stronger legs and improved balance.

INSTRUCTIONS

1. Sit comfortably on a chair, keeping your feet flat on the ground and your spine straight. Engage your core muscles to maintain stability.

2. Slowly lift your left leg, extending it straight out in front of you. If needed, use your hands to support your leg in this extended position.

3. Once your leg is extended, begin to flex your leg up and down at the knee. Perform the desired number of repetitions, keeping your core engaged throughout the movement.

4. After completing the repetitions, gently lower your left leg back to the starting position, placing your foot flat on the ground.

5. Repeat the same sequence of movements with your right leg.

X MISTAKES TO AVOID

- **Rounding the Back:** Ensure your spine remains straight throughout the exercise.

- **Holding Breath:** Breathe consistently throughout the exercise.

- **Using Momentum:** Lift and lower the leg in a controlled manner, avoiding any jerky movements.

FOOT FLEXING

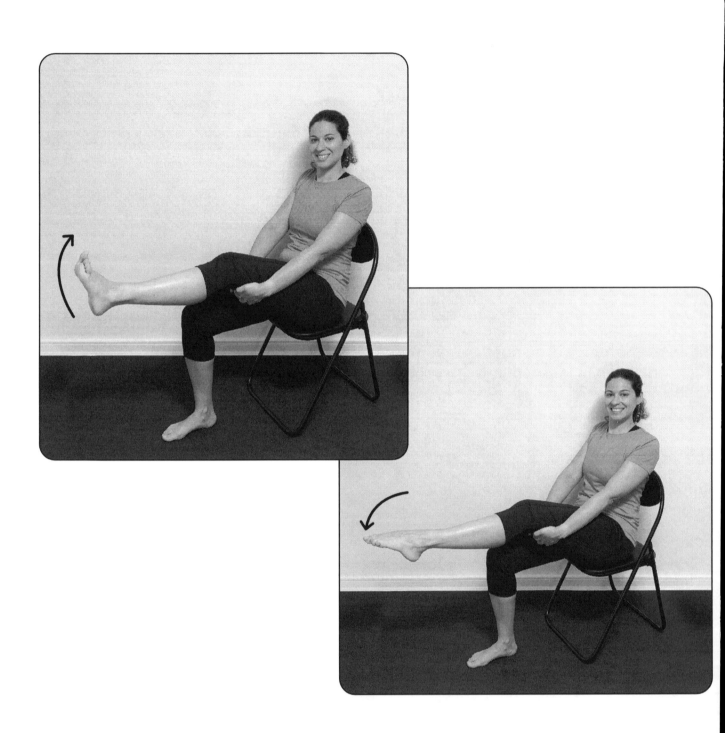

The Chair Flexing Foot Pose is a gentle yet effective way to engage and stretch the muscles of the feet and ankles. By methodically flexing and pointing one foot at a time, practitioners can focus on muscle engagement and flexibility. This pose is particularly beneficial for those who spend long hours sitting, as it helps counteract stiffness in the feet and promotes better circulation. Regular practice can lead to improved foot flexibility and reduced tension in the lower extremities.

INSTRUCTIONS

1. Sit comfortably on a chair, extending your spine and closing your eyes to relax.

2. Raise your left leg to about 40 degrees, keeping your right foot firmly on the floor.

3. While maintaining the leg at a 40-degree angle, move the ankle of the left foot by flexing and pointing the toes.

4. Repeat the flex and point motion a few times.

5. Release the left leg and repeat the same process with the right leg.

✗ MISTAKES TO AVOID

- **Overflexing:** Avoid excessive flexing or pointing, which can strain the foot muscles.

- **Lifting Leg Too High:** Ensure the leg remains at a comfortable angle, around 40 degrees.

- **Rapid Movements:** The flexing of the ankle and toes should be done carefully and in a controlled manner.

CACTUS ARMS

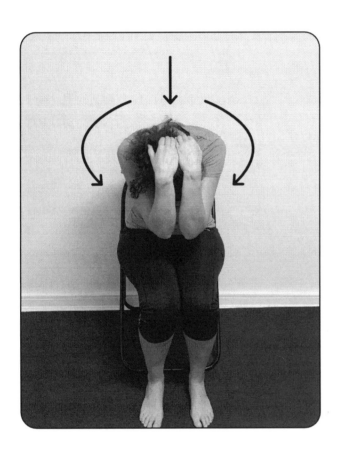 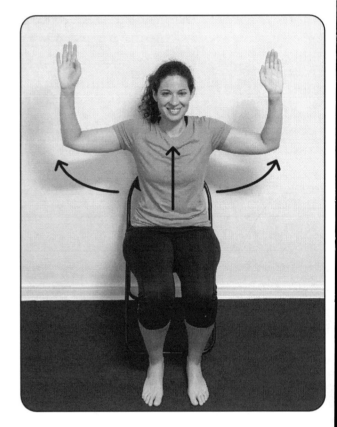

The Cactus Arms pose is a rejuvenating seated exercise that focuses on enhancing the flexibility and strength of the arms and shoulders. By moving the arms in a controlled flow, practitioners can experience improved blood circulation and reduced tension in the upper body.

INSTRUCTIONS

1. Sit comfortably on a chair, ensuring your spine is straight and your feet are flat on the ground.

2. As you inhale, bring your arms to shoulder level, bending at the elbows. Ensure your palms face forward, keeping the forearms perpendicular to the shoulders.

3. Exhale and bring your arms in front, pressing your forearms and palms against each other. While you do this motion, lower your head and hide your face behind the closed arms.

4. Inhale again and extend them out at shoulder level.

5. Repeat multiple times.

✗ MISTAKES TO AVOID

- **Rapid Movements:** Ensure you move your arms in a controlled and deliberate manner, avoiding any jerky motions.

- **Misalignment:** Ensure your arms remain at shoulder level or slightly below when in the cactus position.

- **Holding Breath:** Breathe consistently throughout the pose. Holding your breath can lead to tension.

SAGE TWIST

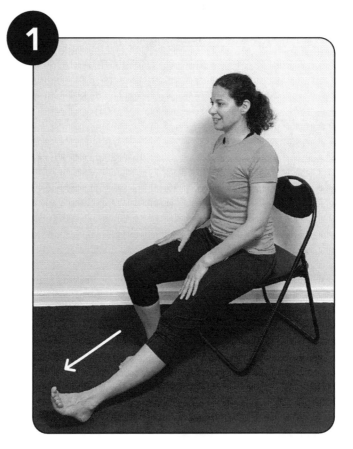

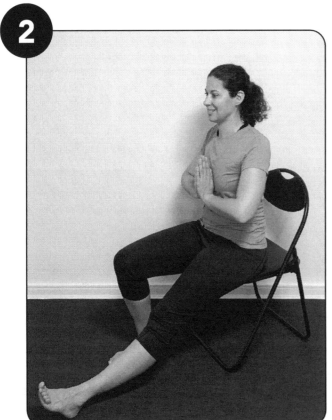

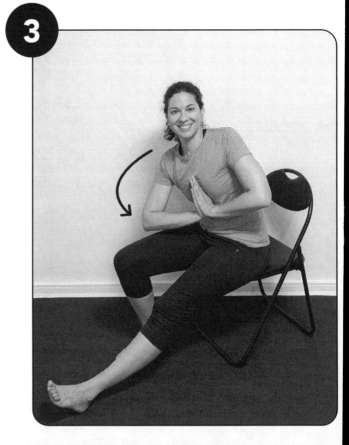

The Sage Twist is a therapeutic seated spinal twist that promotes spinal flexibility. By engaging the core and rotating the spine, it rejuvenates the back muscles, helping to relieve tension and improve posture. In addition, the conscious deep breathing paired with the twist encourages relaxation, stress relief, and enhanced oxygen flow throughout the body.

INSTRUCTIONS

1. Begin by sitting comfortably on a chair with your spine straight and both feet flat on the ground. Extend your left leg forward, ensuring only the heel touches the ground while keeping the right foot flat.

2. As you inhale, bring your palms together in a prayer position in front of your chest.

3. On your exhale, bend slightly forward and twist your torso to the left, aiming to align your prayer hands with the center of your chest. Maintain this position, taking a few deep breaths, allowing the twist to deepen with each exhale.

   On an inhale, slowly return to the starting position.

   Repeat a few times, then do the same on the opposite side.

✗ MISTAKES TO AVOID

- **Over-twisting:** The twist should be gentle and controlled. Avoid straining or pushing too hard to get a deeper twist; this could cause harm to the spine or muscles.

- **Misalignment of Hands:** Ensure that your prayer hands align with the center of your chest during the twist. Avoid letting the hands drift too high or too low.

- **Holding Breath:** Breathing deeply and steadily is crucial. Avoid holding your breath; instead, let your breathing guide and deepen the twist naturally.

- **Rushing Through the Pose:** Take your time to settle into the pose and breathe deeply. Avoid rushing or moving too quickly between positions, as this can reduce the exercise's effectiveness and increase the risk of injury.

REVOLVED POSE

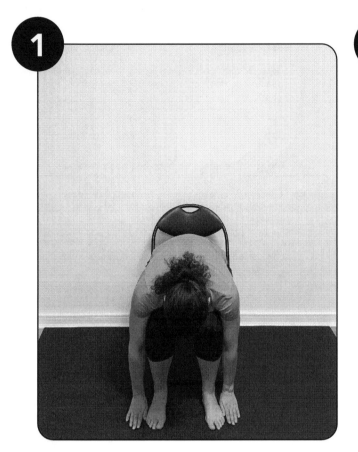

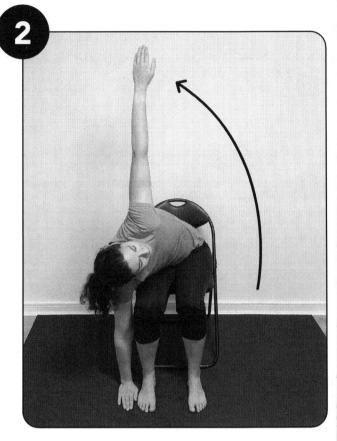

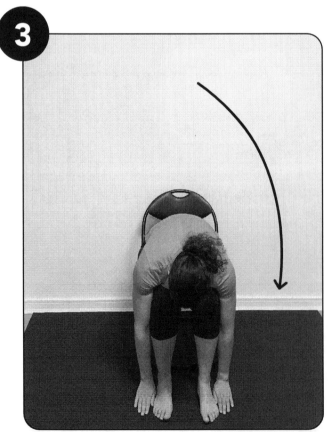

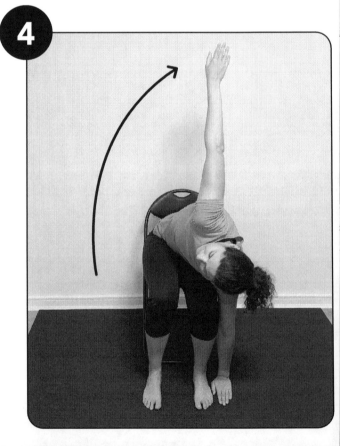

The Revolved Pose is a seated adaptation of the classic twist, designed to offer spinal rejuvenation and waist flexibility. Executed with the support of a chair, it ensures safety and accessibility, making it especially beneficial for those with mobility challenges and yoga beginners. This pose not only enhances spinal health but also aids in digestion and stimulates the abdominal organs.

INSTRUCTIONS

Begin by sitting comfortably on a chair with your spine straight and feet flat on the ground, hip-width apart.

1. As you inhale, lengthen your spine, ensuring your back remains upright. Place your hands beside your feet, reaching for the floor with your palms

2. On the exhale, gently twist your torso to the left side. Raise your left arm upwards while extending it. Simultaneously, turn your head to gaze over your left shoulder, maintaining the twist in your torso and the elevation of your arm. With each breath, aim to deepen the twist slightly, all while keeping your spine straight. Hold this position for approximately 4-6 breaths, feeling the stretch along your spine and the sides of your waist.

3-4. Gradually return to the center by reversing the movements, then repeat the twist on the right side.

✗ MISTAKES TO AVOID

- **Over-Twisting:** Ensure you don't force the twist. Move only as far as your body comfortably allows.

- **Slouching:** Keep your spine straight throughout the pose. Avoid rounding your back.

- **Straining the Neck:** Ensure your neck is in line with your spine. Don't over-rotate it.

BOAT

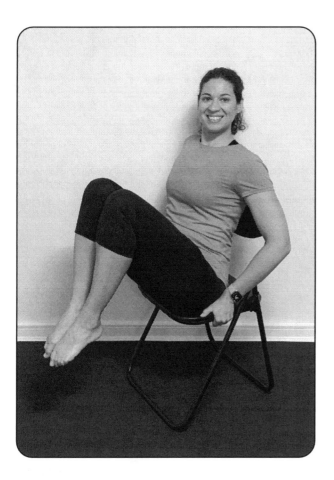

INSTRUCTIONS

1. Ensure you're seated comfortably with your spine elongated.

2. As you inhale, grab the sides of the chair with your hands. Your fingers should curl underneath the chair, with your thumbs resting on top near your buttocks. This grip will provide stability and balance.

3. Exhale and gently lift your feet, keeping your knees bent. For added stability, you can cross your ankles. Ensure your knees align with your chest but maintain some distance from your torso.

4. As you inhale, lengthen your spine and draw your abdomen in. This engagement will help bear the weight of your legs and maintain balance. Your body will naturally lean back, but ensure your chest remains open.

5. Ensure your lower back remains straight. Ground yourself on the chair with your sit bones, even as you lean back and lift your legs. This grounding will help maintain a straight spine.

6. Once you've achieved a comfortable position, hold the pose for 3-4 breaths.

7. To exit the pose, uncross your ankles if they were crossed, and gently place your feet back on the floor. Release your grip on the chair and return to a neutral position.

The Boat pose that challenges core strength and balance while seated. It offers a safer alternative to the traditional yoga boat pose, making it accessible for individuals of various fitness levels. By engaging the core and focusing on breath, this pose fosters stability and concentration.

✗ MISTAKES TO AVOID

- **Overarching the Back:** Ensure your lower back doesn't curve excessively. This can strain the spine and compromise core engagement.

- **Overlifting the Legs:** Avoid lifting your legs too high, which can put undue pressure on the lower back.

MUSCLE TONING EXERCISES

LEG RAISES

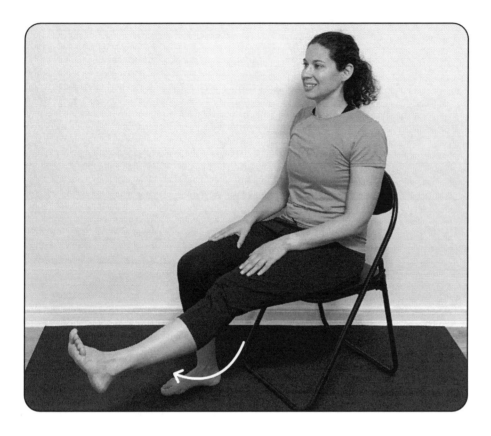

Leg Raises is a simple yet effective movement aimed at strengthening the thigh and hip muscles. Performed while seated, it offers a low-impact way to engage and tone the lower body. Regular practice can enhance leg strength, flexibility, and overall lower body endurance.

INSTRUCTIONS

1. Begin by sitting upright on a chair, ensuring your spine is straight and your feet are flat on the ground, hip-width apart.

2. Draw your abdomen in, engaging your core muscles to provide stability.

3. Slowly lift one leg, keeping it straight, until it's parallel to the ground or as high as comfortably possible.

4. Maintain this position for a couple of breaths, feeling the engagement in your thigh and hip muscles.

5. Gently lower your leg back to the starting position.

6. Perform the same steps with the other leg. Aim for multiple repetitions on each side.

✗ MISTAKES TO AVOID

- **Arching the Back:** Ensure your back remains straight throughout the exercise to avoid strain.

- **Using Momentum:** Avoid using momentum to lift the leg. The movement should be controlled and deliberate.

- **Lifting Too High:** Only lift the leg as high as is comfortable. Overextending can lead to strain.

CHAIR SQUATS

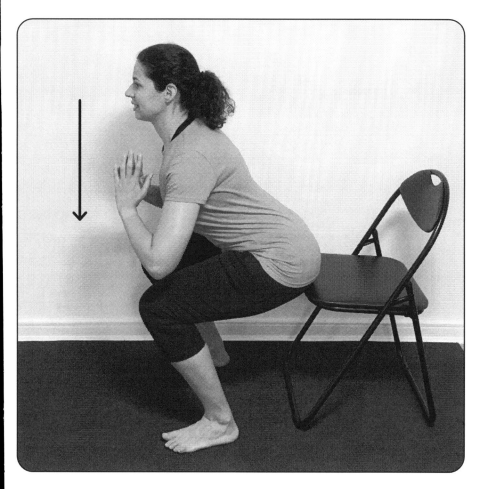

Chair Squats are a foundational exercise designed to target the muscles of the lower body, including the quads, hamstrings, and glutes. By using a chair as a guide, practitioners can ensure proper form and depth. This exercise is especially beneficial for those looking to enhance leg strength, improve balance, and promote functional mobility in daily activities.

INSTRUCTIONS

1. Start by standing upright with a chair positioned behind you. Your feet should be hip-width apart. Ensure the chair is close enough so that when you squat down, your bottom can easily touch its seat.

2. Take a deep breath in, lifting your arms out in front of you for balance.

3. As you exhale, push your hips back and bend your knees, lowering your body towards the chair. Lightly touch the chair with your glutes, but don't sit down.

4. Pause briefly in the squat position, ensuring your knees are aligned with your toes.

5. Push through your heels, straightening your legs, and return to the starting position.

6. Aim for multiple repetitions, gradually increasing as you build strength and endurance.

✗ MISTAKES TO AVOID

- **Knees Over Toes:** Ensure your knees don't extend past your toes when squatting down.

- **Lifting Heels:** Keep your heels firmly planted on the ground as you squat.

CALF RAISES

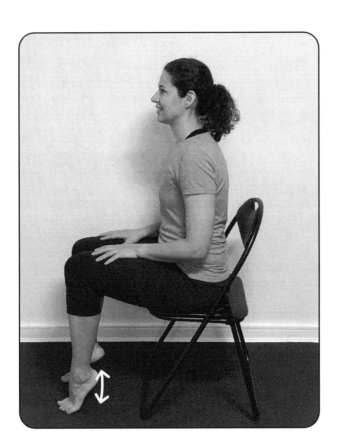

INSTRUCTIONS

1. Begin by sitting upright on a sturdy chair, ensuring your spine is straight and your feet are flat on the ground, hip-width apart.

2. Press down through the balls of your feet and lift your heels off the ground, rising onto your tiptoes.

3. At the peak of the lift, engage your calf muscles, holding the position for a moment.

4. Slowly lower your heels back to the ground in a controlled manner.

5. Aim for multiple repetitions, gradually increasing as you build strength and endurance.

✗ MISTAKES TO AVOID

- **Rapid Movements:** Ensure you lift and lower your heels in a controlled manner, avoiding any jerky motions.

- **Neglecting the Calves:** It's crucial to actively engage the calf muscles during the lift to ensure maximum benefit. One effective method is to hold the position briefly.

The Calf Raises Chair exercise is a straightforward yet effective movement targeting the calf muscles. By lifting onto the tiptoes, practitioners can strengthen and tone the calves, enhancing stability and balance. This exercise is especially beneficial for those looking to improve lower leg strength and can be easily incorporated into daily routines.

ALTERNATIVE CALF RAISES

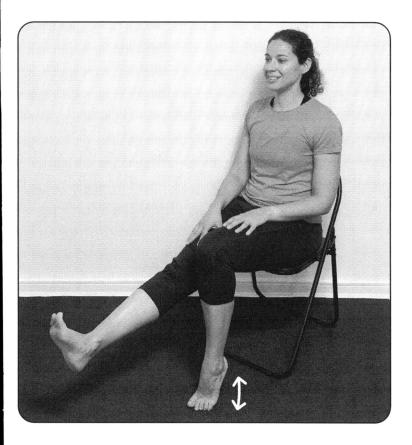

The Alternative Calf Raises is a more challenging version of the calf raises exercise previously proposed. It not only benefits the calves but also targets the thigh and hip muscles of the raised leg. This exercise is especially beneficial for those looking to improve lower leg strength and can be easily incorporated into daily routines.

INSTRUCTIONS

1. Begin by sitting upright on a sturdy chair, ensuring your spine is straight and your feet are flat on the ground, hip-width apart.

2. Slowly lift your right leg, keeping it straight, until it's parallel to the ground or as high as comfortably possible.

3. Press down through the ball of your left foot and lift your heel off the ground, rising onto your tiptoes.

4. At the peak of the lift, engage your calf muscles, holding the position for a moment.

5. Slowly lower your heel back to the ground in a controlled manner.

6. Aim for multiple repetitions, gradually increasing as you build strength and endurance.

✗ MISTAKES TO AVOID

- **Rapid Movements:** Ensure you lift and lower your heels in a controlled manner, avoiding any jerky motions.

- **Neglecting the Calves:** It's crucial to actively engage the calf muscles during the lift to ensure maximum benefit. One effective method is to hold the position briefly.

- **Lowering the Raised Leg:** For maximum results, ensure your raised leg stays parallel to the ground while you perform the exercise.

MOUNTAIN POSE ONE LEG BACKLIFT

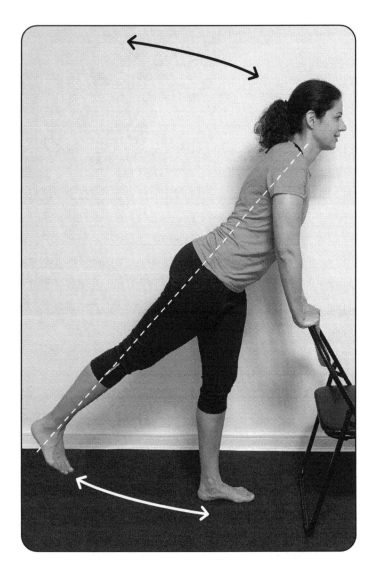

The Mountain Pose Chair One Leg Backlift is a modified standing pose that focuses on strengthening the legs and improving balance. By lifting one leg at a time, it challenges stability and engages the core. This pose is especially beneficial for those looking to enhance their leg strength and hip mobility in a controlled and supported manner.

INSTRUCTIONS

1. Stand in front of a chair, ensuring your feet are hip-width apart and your spine is straight.

2. Slightly bend your torso forward and find your balance by holding onto the chair.

3. Raise one leg backward, keeping it straight.

4. Hold this position briefly, feeling the engagement in the leg and the stretch in the hip flexors.

5. Lower your leg back to the ground, returning to the starting position.

6. Repeat the same steps with the other leg.

✗ MISTAKES TO AVOID

- **Overextending the Leg:** Avoid raising the leg too high, which can strain the lower back.

CHAIR SHUFFLE LEG

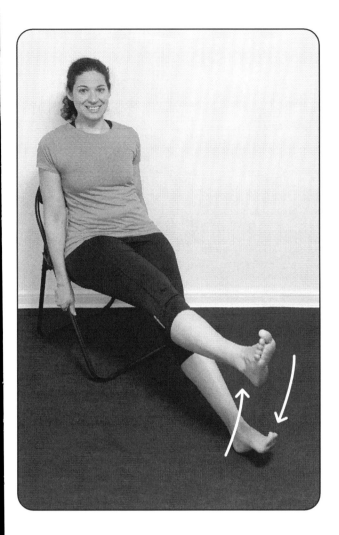

The Chair Leg Shuffle is a seated exercise designed to strengthen the leg muscles, particularly the quadriceps, while also engaging the core for balance and stability. Performed on a chair, it offers a low-impact yet effective workout for individuals of all fitness levels.

INSTRUCTIONS

1. Sit at the edge of a sturdy chair, ensuring your back is erect. Place your hands on either side of the chair for added stability. Gently lean your upper body backward.

2. Extend both legs in front of you, resting only the heels on the ground. Your toes should be pointed upwards, creating a slight angle with your legs.

3. With a controlled motion, elevate one leg, aiming to bring it parallel to the floor or as high as comfortably possible. The opposite leg's heel remains grounded, offering support.

4. Gradually lower the raised leg back to its starting position. Then, lift the other leg in a similar manner. Completing both lifts counts as one full repetition.

✗ MISTAKES TO AVOID

- **Arching the Back:** Ensure you maintain a straight back throughout the exercise, resisting the urge to arch.

- **Rushing the Movement:** The leg lift should be deliberate and controlled. Avoid the temptation to speed through repetitions.

- **Overlifting:** While the goal is to raise the leg parallel to the floor, it's essential to stay within a comfortable range, preventing any strain.

STEP OUT

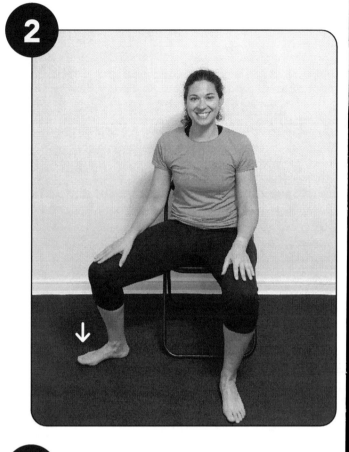

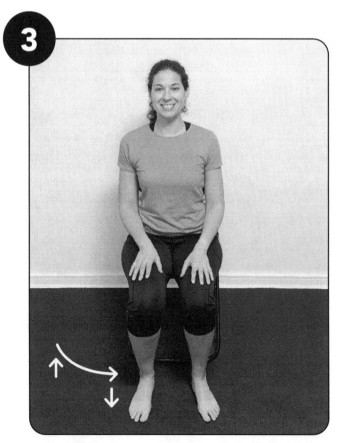

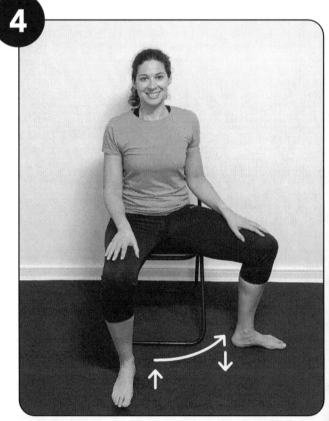

The Step Out Chair exercise is a seated movement designed to engage the muscles of the outer thighs and hips. With this exercise, practitioners can target specific muscle groups, enhancing flexibility and strength. This low-impact exercise is especially beneficial for those looking to improve lower body mobility in a controlled and supported environment.

INSTRUCTIONS

1. Begin by sitting upright on a sturdy chair, ensuring your spine is straight and your feet are flat on the ground, hip-width apart. Lift your right foot off the ground slightly.

2. Gently step your right foot out to the side, extending it as far as comfortably possible while keeping the foot flat.

3. Bring your right foot back to the starting position.

4. Perform the same steps with the left foot. Aim for multiple repetitions on each side.

✗ MISTAKES TO AVOID

- **Leaning Too Much:** Ensure you maintain an upright posture throughout the exercise. Avoid leaning to the opposite side when stepping out.

- **Overextending:** Only step out as far as is comfortable. Overextending can lead to strain or injury.

- **Losing Core Engagement:** Keep the core engaged throughout to maintain stability and protect the lower back.

CURLS

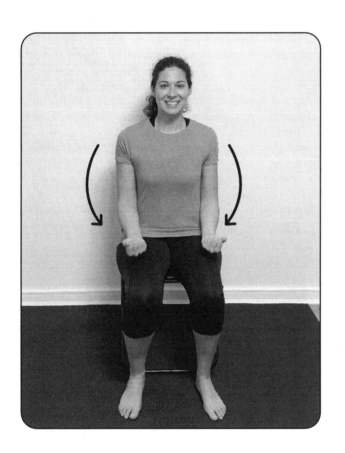 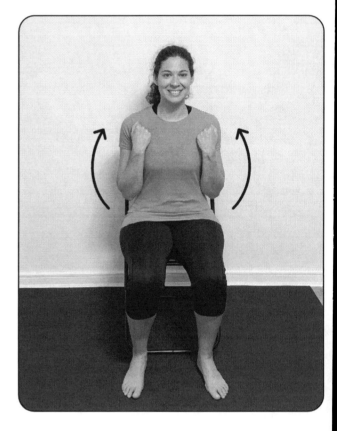

The Curl exercise is a simple seated movement designed to target and strengthen the bicep muscles. By curling the hands towards the shoulders, practitioners can effectively engage the biceps, promoting better arm strength and definition. This exercise is especially beneficial for those looking to enhance arm strength in a controlled and supported setting. Small weights can be used if desired.

INSTRUCTIONS

1. Sit up straight in a chair, ensuring your spine is lengthened. Place your feet flat on the ground, hip-width apart.

2. Extend your arms down by your sides with your palms facing forward.

3. Take a deep breath in, preparing for the movement.

4. As you exhale, bend your elbows and curl your hands up towards your shoulders, keeping your upper arms stationary.

5. At the peak of the curl, engage your bicep muscles, holding the position briefly.

6. Slowly extend your arms back to the starting position.

7. Aim for multiple repetitions, gradually increasing as you build strength.

✗ MISTAKES TO AVOID

- **Using Momentum:** Ensure the curling motion is controlled. Avoid using momentum or swinging your arms.

- **Lifting Shoulders:** Keep your shoulders relaxed and avoid shrugging them during the curl.

SEATED TOE TAPS

LEFT

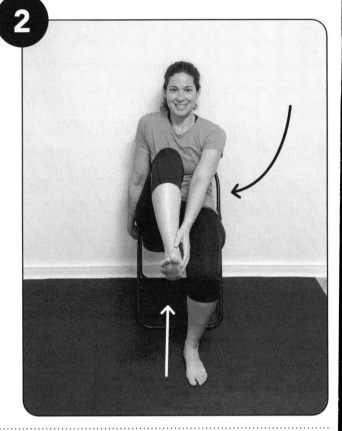

RIGHT

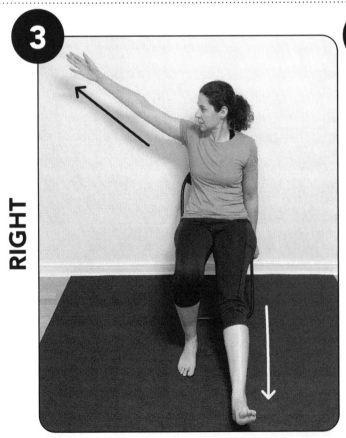

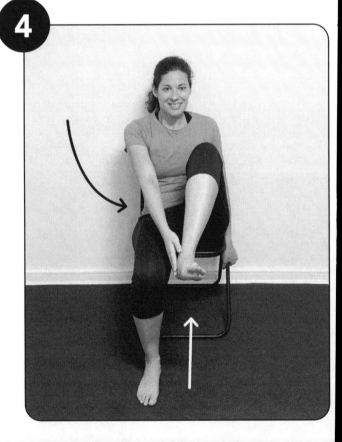

MUSCLE TONING EXERCISES

The Seated Toe Taps exercise helps strengthen your legs and core while sitting. By twisting and reaching, you work on your flexibility and balance. It's a simple way to keep your muscles active and improve co-ordination.

INSTRUCTIONS

1. Begin by sitting upright in a chair. Extend your left arm above shoulder level. Simultaneously, extend your right leg straight out in front of you, keeping your heel in contact with the ground.

2. As you lift your right leg, gently twist your torso to the right. Aim to touch your right foot with your left hand.

   Lower your right leg back down and untwist your torso, returning to the initial position.

   Perform the exercise for multiple repetitions, then switch sides.

3-4. Repeat the above instructions for the other side.

✗ MISTAKES TO AVOID

- **Over-Twisting:** Avoid twisting your torso too aggressively. The movement should be gentle to prevent any strain on the spine.

- **Lifting the Leg Too High:** Ensure you lift the leg to a comfortable height. Overextending can strain the hip flexors. Focus on reaching with your arm.

KNEE TO NOSE

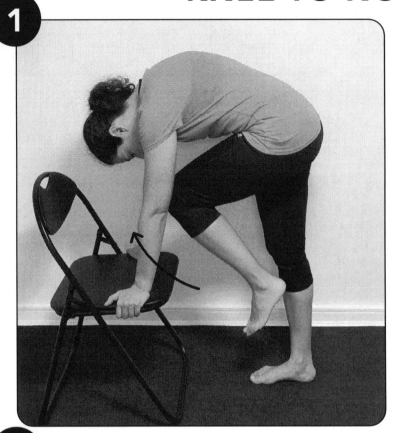

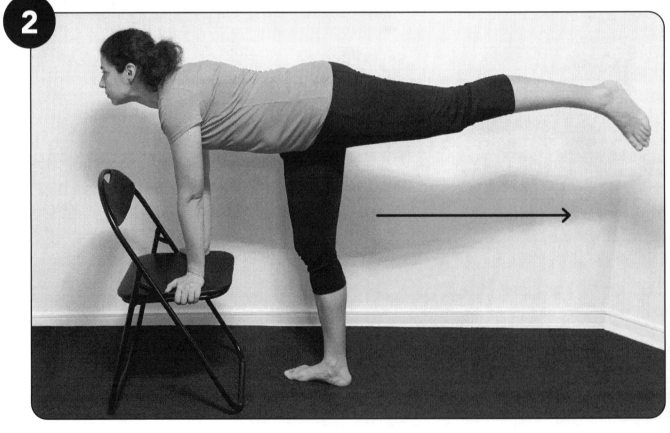

This is a dynamic movement that combines balance, strength, and flexibility. By integrating the breath with motion, this exercise not only enhances leg strength but also promotes mindfulness and coordination. Suitable for individuals of all levels, it's a great way to invigorate the body and refresh the mind during a chair yoga session.

INSTRUCTIONS

Stand in front of a chair with your feet hip-width apart.

Place your hands on the chair for support. As you inhale, stand tall and ensure your spine is straight.

1. On your exhale, bend your left knee and bring it towards your nose.

2. Inhale and extend your left leg out behind you, keeping your foot flexed. Hold the position for a few breaths.

Perform the exercise for multiple repetitions, then switch sides.

✗ MISTAKES TO AVOID

- **Overstretching:** Avoid extending the leg too far back, which can strain the lower back.

- **Losing Balance:** Ensure you maintain a firm grip on the chair to avoid losing balance.

- **Rushing the Movement:** Move slowly and deliberately, coordinating each movement with your breath.

- **Not Engaging Core:** Engage your core muscles throughout the exercise for stability and to protect your lower back.

LEG PUSH-UP

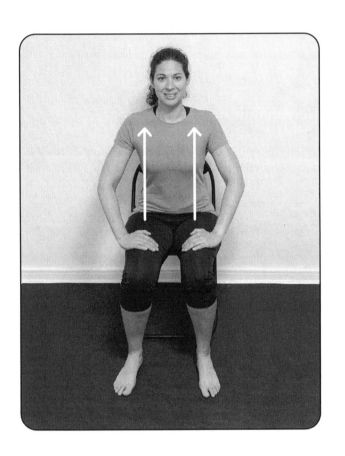 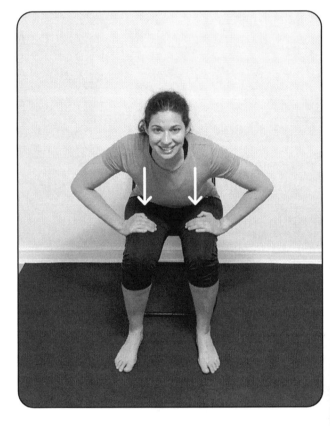

The Leg Push Up is a seated exercise that focuses on strengthening the arms, shoulders, and chest while also engaging the core for stability. It offers a unique way to work on the upper body muscles without the need for any additional equipment, making it ideal for those looking for an effective yet simple workout.

INSTRUCTIONS

1. Sit comfortably on a chair, positioning your legs slightly wider than hip-width apart. Ensure your feet are flat on the ground.

2. Rest your hands atop your knees, palms facing down.

3. With a straight back, lean your chest forward towards your legs, going as low as you comfortably can.

4. Engage your arms and shoulders to push yourself back to the upright starting position.

5. Continue the movement for the desired number of repetitions.

✗ MISTAKES TO AVOID

- **Curved Back:** It's essential to keep the back straight throughout the movement. Avoid rounding or arching the back.

- **Shifting Hand Position:** Keep your hands firmly on your knees throughout the exercise. Avoid letting them slide or reposition.

STANDING HAMSTRING CURL

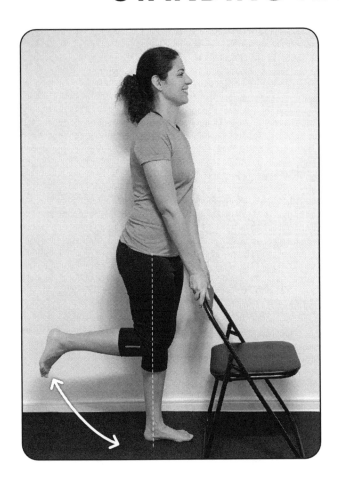

INSTRUCTIONS

1. Begin by standing upright behind a chair, placing both hands on the backrest for support. Your feet should be hip-width apart with your posture straight.

2. Bend your right knee and lift your right heel towards your buttocks. Keep the thighs aligned and close together.

3. At the peak of the lift, engage your hamstring muscles, holding the position for a moment.

4. Slowly extend your right leg back to the starting position in a controlled manner.

5. Perform the same steps with the left leg. Aim for multiple repetitions on each side.

✗ MISTAKES TO AVOID

- **Arching the Back:** Ensure your back remains straight throughout the exercise to avoid strain.

- **Swinging the Leg:** The movement should be controlled and deliberate. Avoid using momentum to lift the leg.

- **Lifting the Thigh:** Ensure the thighs remain aligned and close together, avoiding any outward movement of the lifting leg.

The Standing Hamstring Curl is a targeted movement designed to engage and strengthen the hamstring muscles. By lifting the heel towards the buttocks, practitioners can effectively work the back of the thigh. This exercise is especially beneficial for those looking to enhance hamstring strength and flexibility in a controlled and supported environment.

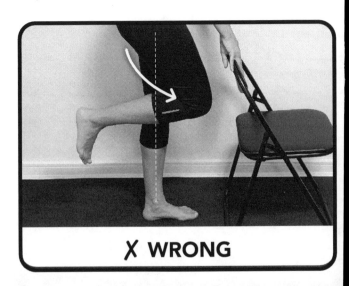

✗ WRONG

CARDIO EXERCISES

SEATED KICK AND PUNCH

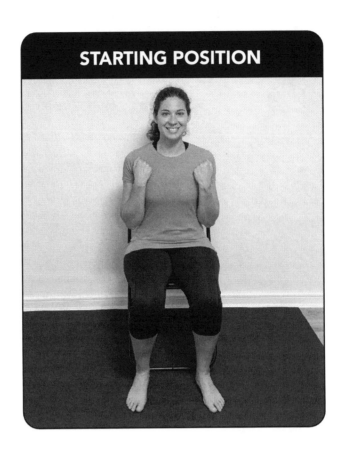

STARTING POSITION

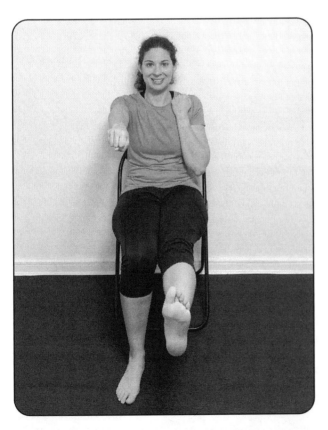

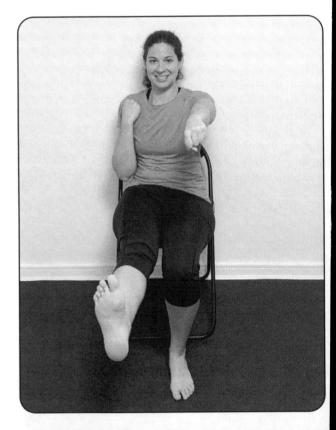

Seated Kicks and Punches is a dynamic chair exercise that combines lower and upper body movements. By integrating kicks with punches, this routine offers a full-body workout that enhances coordination, strength, and cardiovascular endurance. Suitable for individuals of all levels, it's a great way to add energy and vigor to any seated exercise session.

INSTRUCTIONS

1. Begin by sitting comfortably on a chair with your spine straight, feet flat on the ground, and hands in loose fists by your sides. Ensure your shoulders are relaxed.

2. Extend your right leg forward in a controlled kick, keeping your foot flexed. Simultaneously, punch forward with your left arm, extending it fully.

3. Retract your left arm and place your right foot back on the ground.

4. Repeat the kick with your left leg and punch with your right arm.

5. Perform this alternating sequence for a set number of repetitions or for a specific duration.

✗ MISTAKES TO AVOID

- **Overextending:** Avoid kicking or punching too forcefully, which can strain muscles.

- **Slouching:** Ensure your spine remains straight throughout the exercise. Avoid leaning back or forward.

- **Holding Breath:** Breathe consistently throughout the movement, coordinating each kick and punch with your breath.

- **Misaligned Shoulders:** Keep your shoulders relaxed and avoid raising them during the punches.

SEATED MARCH

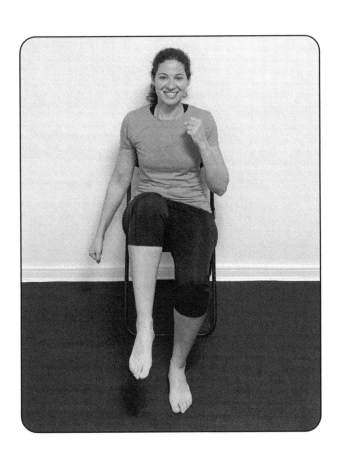 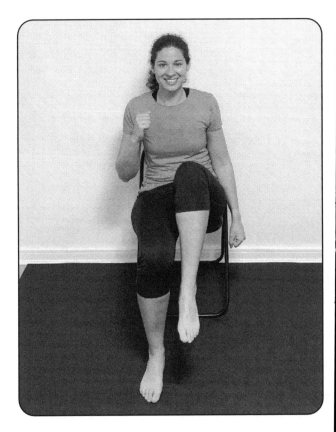

The Seated March is a simple yet effective chair exercise that targets the lower body and core. By mimicking the motion of marching while seated, it offers a low-impact cardiovascular workout that can be easily incorporated into daily routines. Suitable for individuals of all fitness levels, the Seated March is a great way to boost circulation and strengthen leg muscles without the need for standing or extensive space.

INSTRUCTIONS

1. Begin by sitting comfortably on a chair with your spine straight, feet flat on the ground, and hands resting on your thighs or by your sides.

2. As you lift your right knee towards your chest, swing your left arm forward in a controlled manner, similar to a marching motion.

3. Gently lower your right foot back to the ground and bring your left arm back to its starting position.

4. Now, as you lift your left knee towards your chest, swing your right arm forward.

5. Gently lower your left foot back to the ground and return your right arm to its starting position.

6. Alternate between the right and left legs, mimicking a marching motion while seated, and coordinating with the opposite arm.

7. Continue this marching sequence for a set number of repetitions or for a specific duration, maintaining a steady rhythm.

✗ MISTAKES TO AVOID

- **Leaning Back:** Ensure you maintain an upright posture throughout the exercise. Avoid leaning back when lifting your knees.

- **Lifting Too High:** Only lift your knee as high as is comfortable, avoiding any strain on the hip or lower back.

TORSO TWIST

1

2

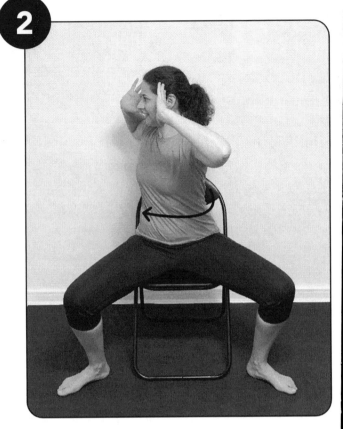

3

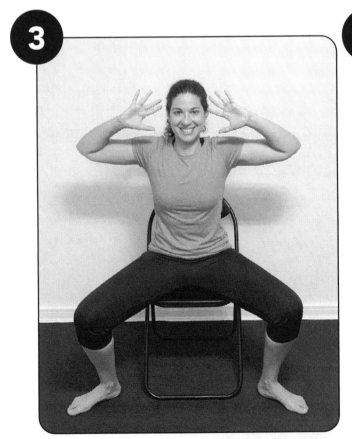

4

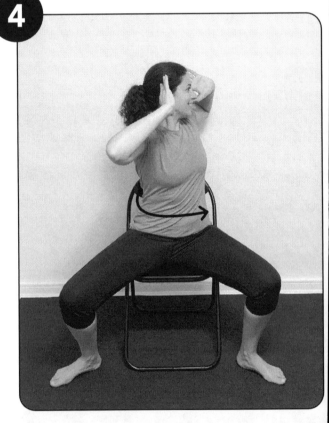

The Torso Twist is a dynamic seated exercise that targets the core muscles, especially the obliques. By incorporating a rhythmic twisting motion, it not only strengthens the midsection but also offers a cardiovascular boost. This exercise is ideal for those looking to enhance core stability, improve spinal flexibility, and add a cardio element to their seated workout routine.

INSTRUCTIONS

1. Begin by sitting comfortably on a chair with your spine straight and feet flat on the ground, hip-width apart.Place both hands on the sides or behind your head, with elbows pointing outwards. Open your legs to ensure balance during the exercise.

2. Twist your torso to the left, ensuring your hips remain stationary and facing forward.

3. Return to the center position.

4. Twist your torso to the left, again making sure your hips stay stationary.

   Continue this alternating twisting sequence for a set number of repetitions or for a specific duration, maintaining a steady rhythm.

✗ MISTAKES TO AVOID

- **Over-Twisting:** Avoid forcing the twist; move only as far as your body comfortably allows.

- **Moving the Hips:** Ensure your hips remain stationary throughout the exercise to isolate the movement to the torso.

- **Straining the Neck:** Keep your neck in line with your spine. Avoid over-rotating it or pressing your head with your hands.

- **Holding Breath:** Breathe consistently throughout the movement, coordinating each twist with your breath.

L AND KICK

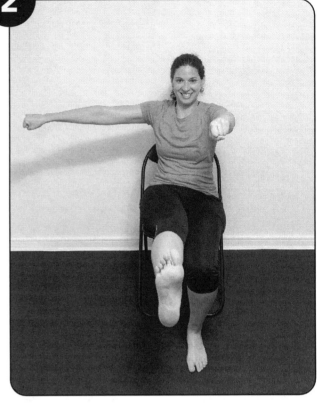

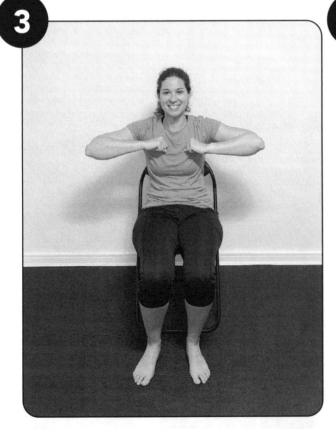

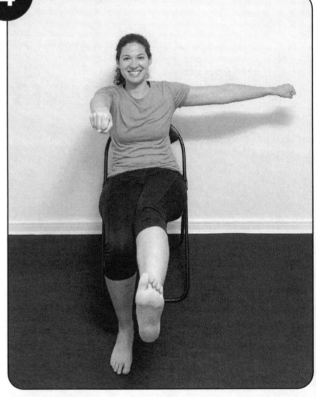

The L and Kick exercise is a unique seated exercise that synergizes upper and lower body movements. By pairing leg kicks with "L" shaped arm movements, this routine offers a comprehensive workout that enhances coordination, strength, and cardiovascular endurance. Ideal for individuals of all fitness levels, it introduces a dynamic twist to traditional seated exercises.

INSTRUCTIONS

1. Start by sitting comfortably in a chair with your spine straight and feet flat on the ground. Begin with your hands formed into fists at your chest, keeping your elbows positioned outside.

2. Extend your right leg forward in a controlled kick. At the same time, extend your right arm to the side and your left arm forward, creating an "L" shape with your arms.

3. Lower your right leg back to the starting position while retracting your arms.

4. Perform the kick with your left leg while forming the "L" shape with your arms in the opposite direction (left arm to the side, right arm forward).

   Continue alternating between these movements for a set number of repetitions or a specific duration.

✗ MISTAKES TO AVOID

- **Incomplete L Shape:** Ensure one arm is fully extended to the side and the other is forward to form a clear "L" shape.

- **Overextending the Kick:** Avoid kicking too high or forcefully, which can strain the hip flexors.

- **Slouching:** Maintain an upright posture throughout the exercise to engage the core properly.

- **Holding Breath:** Breathe consistently throughout the movement, coordinating each kick and arm movement with your breath.

CROSS PUNCHES

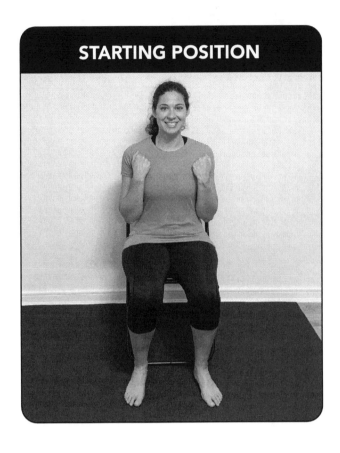

STARTING POSITION

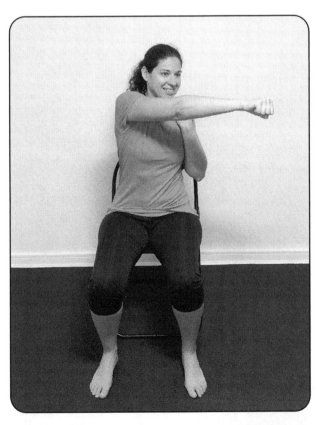

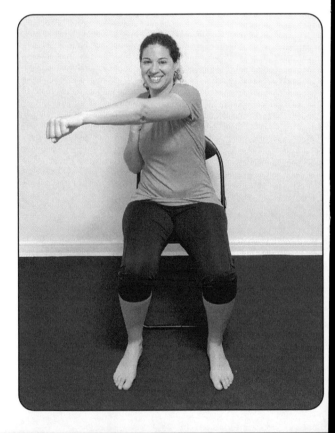

Cross Punches are a dynamic exercise that combines strength, coordination, and aerobic activity. By delivering powerful punches across the body, participants not only engage the arms but also the core and oblique muscles. This movement offers a full-body workout, enhancing cardiovascular health, muscle tone, and overall agility. Whether you're looking to boost your fitness level or add some energy to your routine, Cross Punches are a versatile and effective choice.

INSTRUCTIONS

1. Stand with your feet shoulder-width apart, keep your knees slightly bent, and raise your hands to shoulder level, assuming a guard position. Spread your legs to improve stability

2. Extend your right arm diagonally across your body, aiming to punch towards the left side, while rotating your torso slightly to the left.

3. Retract your right arm back to the guard position.

4. Extend your left arm diagonally across your body, aiming to punch towards the right side, while rotating your torso slightly to the right.

5. Continue this alternating cross-punching motion in a rhythmic manner for a set number of repetitions or for a specific duration.

✗ MISTAKES TO AVOID

- **Overextending the Arm:** Ensure you don't lock out your elbow when punching to avoid strain or injury.

- **Holding Breath:** Breathe consistently throughout the movement, coordinating each punch with your breath.

- **Not Engaging the Core:** Ensure you're engaging your core muscles throughout to stabilize your movements and add power to your punches.

STARS

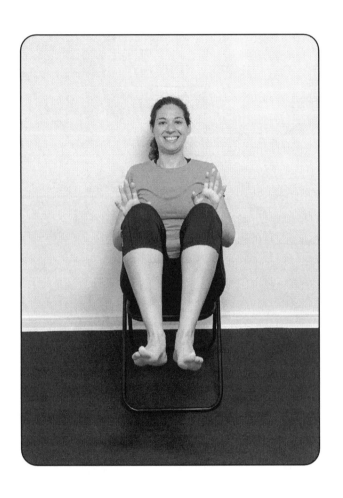 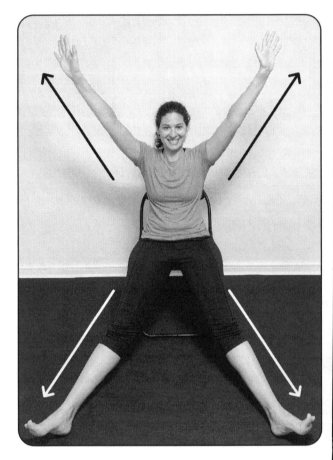

The Stars exercise offers a seated variation of the traditional star jumps, providing an opportunity for cardiovascular engagement without the need to stand. By extending the arms and legs in a star-like motion from a seated position, participants can elevate their heart rate, enhance coordination, and engage multiple muscle groups. This exercise is perfect for those seeking a low-impact yet effective cardio workout, promoting endurance, agility, and overall fitness from the comfort of a chair.

INSTRUCTIONS

1. Begin from a variation of the boat position, with your feet lifted off the floor and your wrists resting on your knees. Find your balance in this position.

2. Inhale as you simultaneously extend your legs, touching the ground with your heels while raising both arms overhead, forming an "X" shape with your body.

3. Exhale as you return to the previous position, bringing your knees back to your chest and lowering your arms to your thighs.

4. Continue this star-like motion in a rhythmic manner for a specified number of repetitions or a set duration.

X MISTAKES TO AVOID

- **Incomplete Movements:** Ensure you fully extend your arms and legs during each motion to maximize the exercise's benefits.

- **Holding Breath:** Breathe consistently throughout the movement, coordinating each star motion with your breath.

- **Not Engaging the Core:** Ensure you're engaging your core muscles throughout to stabilize your movements and protect your lower back.

- **Rushing:** Avoid rushing the transition from a boat position to an X position. Take the time to find your balance, as rushing can lead to injuries and won't effectively engage your core.

UPPERCUTS

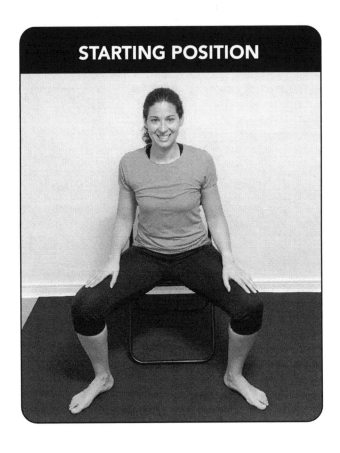

STARTING POSITION

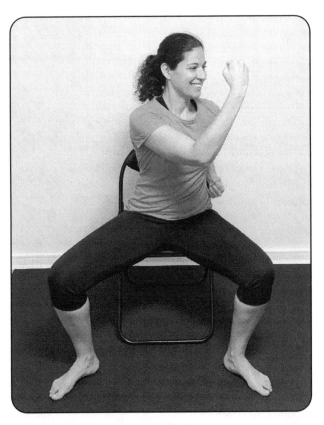

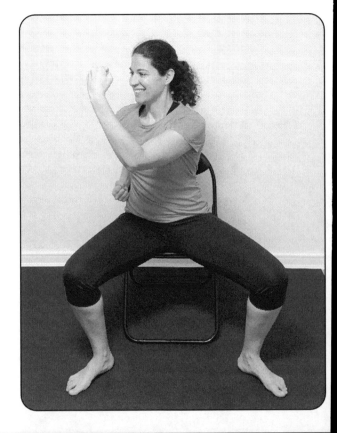

The Uppercuts exercise offers a dynamic upper body workout from a seated position, drawing inspiration from boxing techniques. By performing controlled uppercut motions, participants can engage their arm and shoulder muscles, while also benefiting from improved coordination and reflexes. This exercise is perfect for those seeking a unique and effective upper body workout that combines strength, agility, and cardiovascular benefits, all from the comfort of a chair.

INSTRUCTIONS

1. Sit comfortably on a chair with your feet flat on the ground, hip-width apart. Engage your core muscles and ensure your shoulders are relaxed.

2. Clench your hands into fists and place them in front of your face, elbows bent and close to your ribcage.

3. Perform an uppercut motion with your right fist, driving it upwards and slightly forward as if aiming for an imaginary target in front of your chin. Your elbow should remain bent, and your arm should move in a tight, controlled arc.

4. Swiftly return your right fist to the starting position.

5. Now perform the uppercut motion with your left fist.

6. Continue alternating uppercuts with each arm in a rhythmic manner for a set number of repetitions or for a specific duration.

✗ MISTAKES TO AVOID

- **Overextending Arms:** Ensure you keep a slight bend in your elbows even at the peak of the uppercut motion to avoid straining the joints.

- **Holding Breath:** Breathe consistently throughout the movement, coordinating each uppercut with your breath.

BUTTERFLY

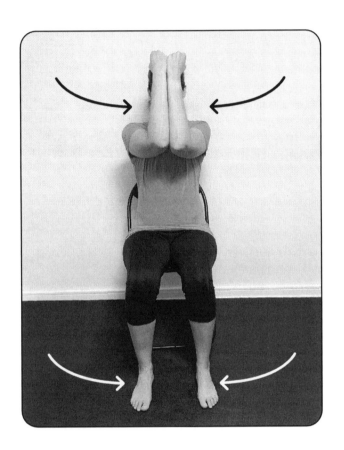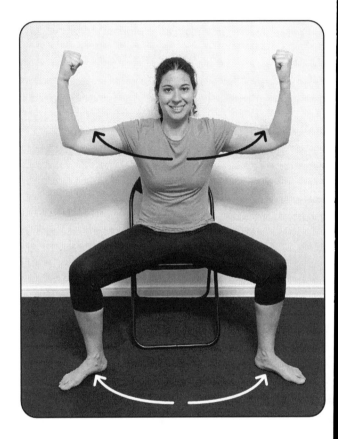

The Butterfly exercise offers a dynamic combination of upper body and thigh movements from a seated position. By simultaneously arms and legs, participants can engage multiple muscle groups, promoting better posture, flexibility, and cardiovascular health. This exercise is perfect for those seeking a comprehensive workout that targets both the upper body and lower body, all while seated comfortably on a chair.

INSTRUCTIONS

1. Sit comfortably on a chair with your feet flat on the ground, hip-width apart.

2. Bend both elbows to approximately 90 degrees, forming fists at head level to cover your face. This position resembles cactus arms but with closed fists.

3. Simultaneously open and close your arms and legs, maintaining the same angle in your knees and arms.

4. Continue this rhythmic open-close motion for a set number of repetitions or a specific duration.

✗ MISTAKES TO AVOID

- **Holding Breath:** Breathe consistently throughout the movement, coordinating each opening with your breath.

- **Rapid Movements:** Focus on controlled, deliberate movements rather than speed to ensure proper muscle engagement.

- **Elbows:** Keep your arms "cactus pose" throughout the exercise.

STEP OUT AND PRESS

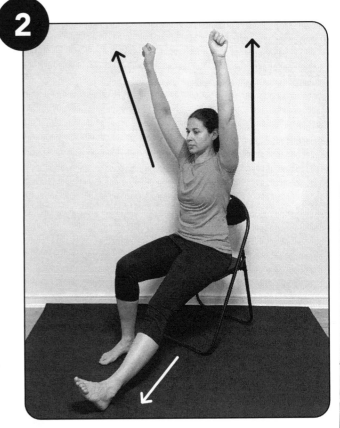

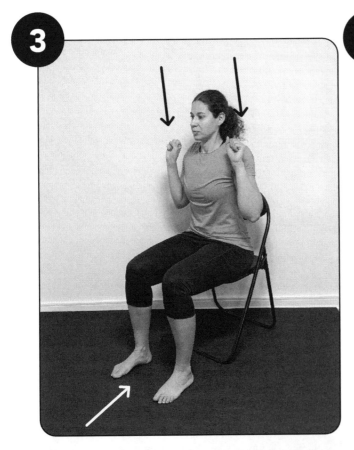

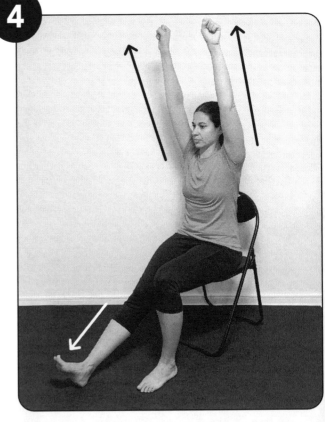

This exercise offers a harmonious blend of arm and leg movements, promoting coordination and balance. As participants extend their limbs, they engage multiple muscle groups, enhancing flexibility and strength. The seated position ensures stability, making it suitable for individuals of various fitness levels.

INSTRUCTIONS

1. Sit comfortably on a chair, ensuring your spine is erect and your shoulders are relaxed and lowered. Bend your elbows and position your hands at shoulder level, keeping them close to your body.

2. Simultaneously extend your arms straight above your head and step one foot forward, fully extending the leg in front of you.

3. Retract your extended leg and arms, returning to the initial position.

4. Repeat the movement, this time extending the opposite leg.

✗ MISTAKES TO AVOID

- **Slouching:** Ensure you maintain an upright posture throughout the exercise.

- **Overextending:** Avoid locking the elbows or knees when extending the arms and legs.

- **Rushing the Movement:** Ensure each movement is controlled and synchronized with your breath.

FLOWS AND ROUTINES

Welcome to the Flow and Routines chapter, where we delve into curated sequences of yoga positions and exercises tailored especially for beginners and seniors. Our primary aim is to enhance mobility and encourage weight loss, ensuring a healthier and more active lifestyle. While we provide recommendations on repetitions, hold times, and overall execution duration, it's essential to remember that these are merely guidelines. Every individual's journey is unique, and we encourage you to adjust these sequences to align with your comfort and fitness level. Listen to your body, and let it guide you through each routine.

SUN SALUTATION

DURATION:
3 min

GOAL:
Relaxation
and Stretching

START

1. PRAYER POSE
(PAGE 14)

2.   HANDS UP
(PAGE 22)

FOLD POSE
(PAGE 17)

**LOW LUNGE ALTER-
NATE LEGS** (PAGE 18)

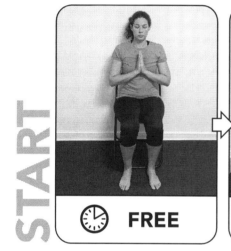

FREE

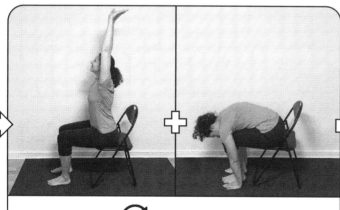

6 reps

3.   HANDS UP
(PAGE 22)

FOLD POSE
(PAGE 17)

4. PRAYER POSE
(PAGE 14)

FINISH

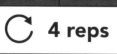

4 reps

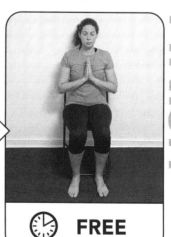

FREE

GENTLE WARM UP

DURATION:
4 min

GOAL:
Flexibility and
Stretching

START

1. SIDE STRETCH LEFT
(PAGE 32)

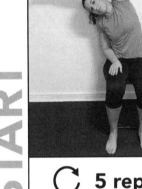

↻ 5 reps

2. SIDE STRETCH RIGHT
(PAGE 32)

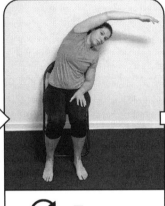

↻ 5 reps

3. SIDE TWIST LEFT AND RIGHT (PAGE 16)

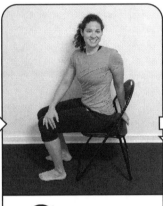

↻ 3 reps

4. CAT-COW POSITION
(PAGE 34)

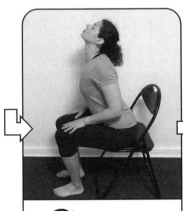

↻ 5 reps

5. SHOULDER CIRCLES
(PAGE 15)

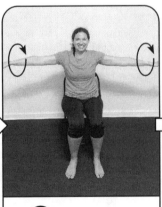

🕐 30 sec

6. CACTUS ARMS
(PAGE 40)

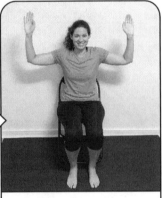

↻ 8 reps

FINISH

BACK PAIN RELIEF

 DURATION:
5 min

 GOAL:
Pain Relief and Mobility

1. CAT-COW POSITION
(PAGE 34)

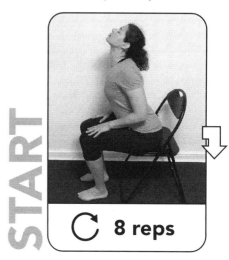

START

 8 reps

2. COBRA POSE
(PAGE 19)

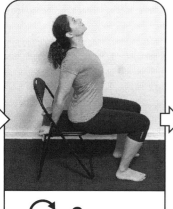

 3 reps

3. SIDE TWIST LEFT AND RIGHT (PAGE 16)

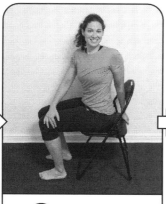

 3 reps

4. SAGE TWIST RIGHT
(PAGE 42)

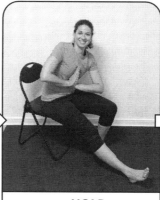

HOLD
15 sec

5. SAGE TWIST LEFT
(PAGE 42)

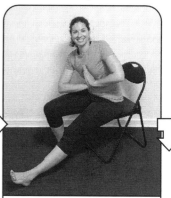

HOLD
15 sec

6. COBRA POSE
(PAGE 19)

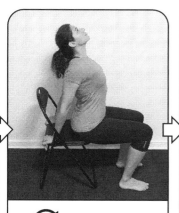

 3 reps

7.   HANDS UP
(PAGE 22)

FOLD POSE
(PAGE 17)

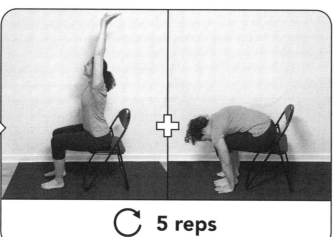

FINISH

 5 reps

NECK AND SHOULDERS RELIEF

⏱ DURATION:
5 min

◎ GOAL:
Pain Relief and Mobility

START

1. SUN BREATHS
(PAGE 26)

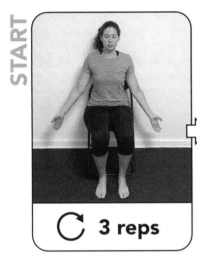

↻ **3 reps**

2. NECK ROLLS
(PAGE 28)

🕐 **40 sec**

3. NECK ROLLS UP & DOWN (PAGE 30)

↻ **5 reps**

4. SHOULDER CIRCLES
(PAGE 15)

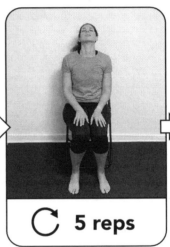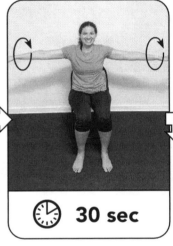

🕐 **30 sec**

5.   HANDS UP
(PAGE 22)

FOLD POSE
(PAGE 17)

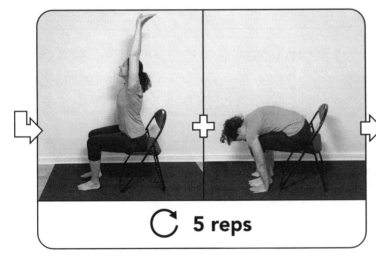

↻ **5 reps**

6. CACTUS ARMS
(PAGE 40)

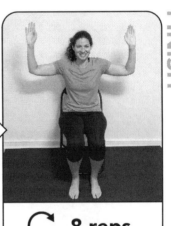

FINISH

↻ **8 reps**

LEGS RELIEF

⏱ DURATION:

3 min

◎ GOAL:

Pain Relief and Mobility

1. LOW LUNGE LEFT
(PAGE 18)

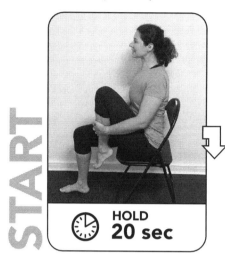

START

🕐 HOLD **20 sec**

2. LOW LUNGE RIGHT
(PAGE 18)

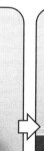

🕐 HOLD **20 sec**

3. ONE-LEGGED SFB LEFT (PAGE 20)

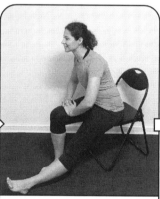

🕐 HOLD **15 sec**

4. ONE-LEGGED SFB RIGHT (PAGE 20)

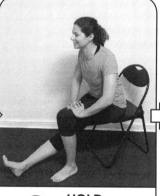

🕐 HOLD **15 sec**

5. PIGEON STRETCH LEFT (PAGE 21)

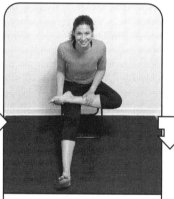

🕐 HOLD **15 sec**

6. PIGEON STRETCH RIGHT (PAGE 21)

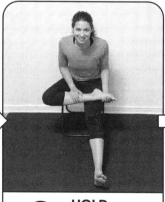

🕐 HOLD **15 sec**

7. FOOT FLEXING LEFT (PAGE 38)

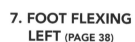

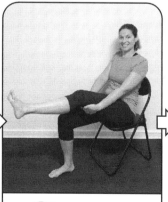

↻ **8 reps**

8. FOOT FLEXING RIGHT (PAGE 38)

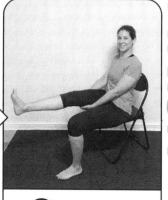

FINISH

↻ **8 reps**

STATIC TONING 1

DURATION:
5 min

GOAL:
Muscle Toning

START

1. PRAYER POSE
(PAGE 14)

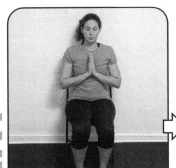

🕐 **FREE**

2. SUN BREATHS
(PAGE 26)

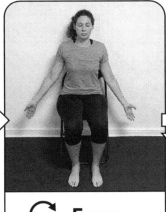

↻ **5 reps**

3. ASSISTED LEG EXTENSIONS LEFT (PAGE 36)

↻ **8 reps**

4. ASSISTED LEG EXTENSIONS RIGHT (PAGE 36)

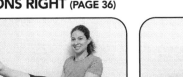

↻ **8 reps**

5. SAGE TWIST RIGHT
(PAGE 42)

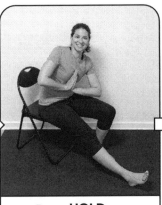

🕐 **HOLD 15 sec**

6. SAGE TWIST LEFT
(PAGE 42)

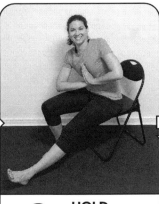

🕐 **HOLD 15 sec**

7. BOAT
(PAGE 46)

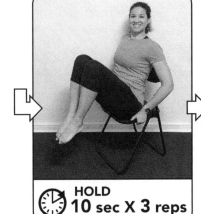

🕐 **HOLD 10 sec X 3 reps**

8. WARRIOR POSE LEFT (PAGE 24)

🕐 **HOLD 15 sec**

9. WARRIOR POSE RIGHT (PAGE 24)

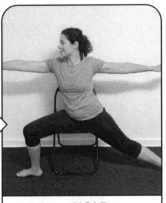

🕐 **HOLD 15 sec**

FINISH

STATIC TONING 2

START

1. PRAYER POSE
(PAGE 14)

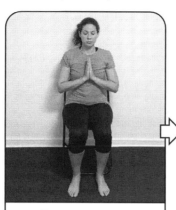

FREE

2. HUMBLE WARRIOR POSE LEFT (PAGE 25)

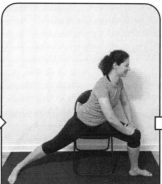

HOLD **15 sec**

3. HUMBLE WARRIOR POSE RIGHT (PAGE 25)

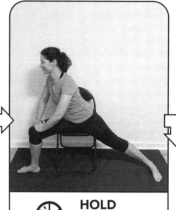

HOLD **15 sec**

4. WARRIOR POSE LEFT (PAGE 24)

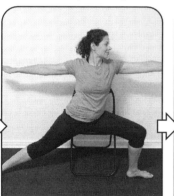

HOLD **15 sec**

5. WARRIOR POSE RIGHT (PAGE 24)

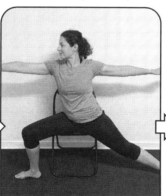

HOLD **15 sec**

6. BOAT (PAGE 46)

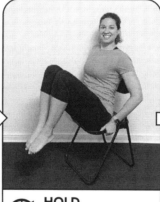

HOLD **10 sec X 3 reps**

7. SAGE TWIST RIGHT (PAGE 42)

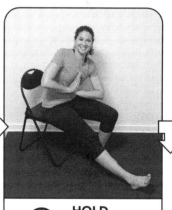

HOLD **15 sec**

8. SAGE TWIST LEFT (PAGE 42)

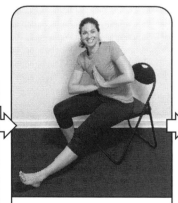

HOLD **15 sec**

9. HIGH LUNGE LEFT (PAGE 23)

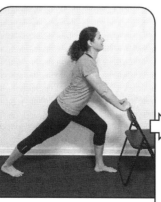

HOLD **20 sec**

10. HIGH LUNGE RIGHT (PAGE 23)

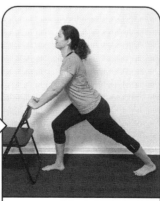

HOLD **20 sec**

FINISH

LEGS TONING 1

⏱ **DURATION:**
4 min

🎯 **GOAL:**
Muscle Toning

1. SEATED MARCH
(PAGE 68)

2. LEG RAISES LEFT
(PAGE 48)

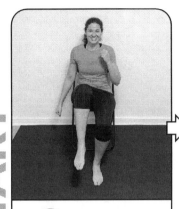
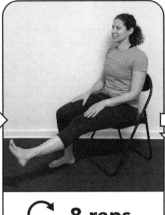

START

🕐 **30 sec**

↻ **8 reps**

3. LEG RAISES RIGHT
(PAGE 48)

4. CALF RAISES
(PAGE 50)

5. ALTERNATIVE CALF RAISES LEFT (PAGE 51)

6. ALTERNATIVE CALF RAISES RIGHT (PAGE 51)

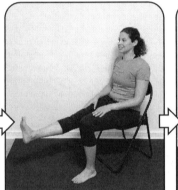
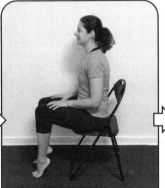
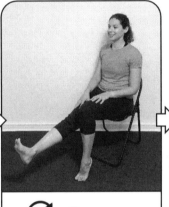
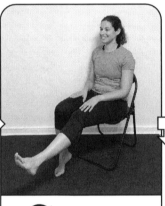

↻ **8 reps**

↻ **10 reps**

↻ **8 reps**

↻ **8 reps**

7. STEP OUT LEFT
(PAGE 54)

8. STEP OUT RIGHT
(PAGE 54)

9. SEATED MARCH
(PAGE 68)

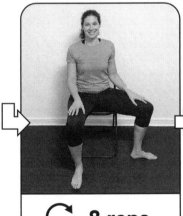
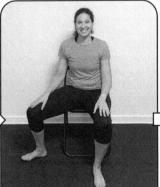
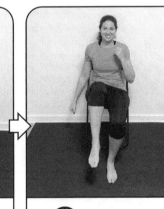

FINISH

↻ **8 reps**

↻ **8 reps**

🕐 **30 sec**

LEGS TONING 2

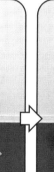

DURATION:
5 min

GOAL:
Muscle Toning

1. SEATED MARCH
(PAGE 68)

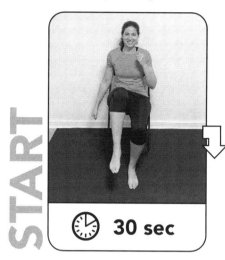

START

🕐 **30 sec**

---

2. STEP OUT LEFT
(PAGE 54)

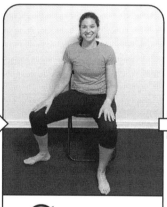

↻ **8 reps**

3. STEP OUT RIGHT
(PAGE 54)

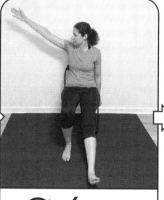

↻ **8 reps**

4. SEATED TOE TAPS ALTERNATE (PAGE 58)

↻ **6 reps per leg**

5. CHAIR SQUATS
(PAGE 49)

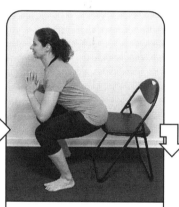

↻ **5 reps**

---

6. STANDING HAM-STRING CURL LEFT (P. 64)

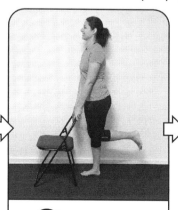

↻ **15 reps**

7. STANDING HAM-STRING CURL RIGHT (P. 64)

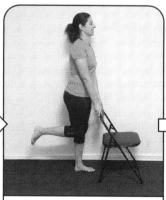

↻ **15 reps**

8. SEATED MARCH
(PAGE 68)

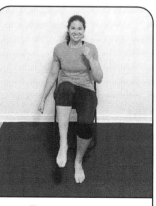

FINISH

🕐 **30 sec**

LEGS TONING 3

 DURATION:

3 min

GOAL:

Muscle Toning

1. SEATED MARCH
(PAGE 68)

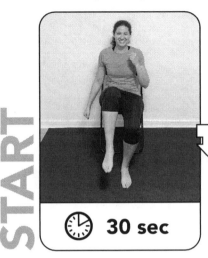

START

⏱ **30 sec**

---

2. CHAIR SHUFFLE LEG
(PAGE 53)

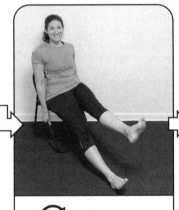

↻ **8 reps***

3. LEG RAISES LEFT
(PAGE 48)

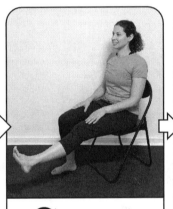

↻ **8 reps**

4. LEG RAISES RIGHT
(PAGE 48)

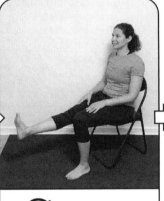

↻ **8 reps**

5. CHAIR SQUATS
(PAGE 49)

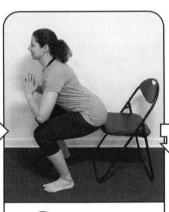

↻ **5 reps**

---

6. MOUNTAIN POSE OLB LEFT (PAGE 52)

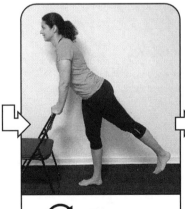

↻ **8 reps**

7. MOUNTAIN POSE OLB RIGHT (PAGE 52)

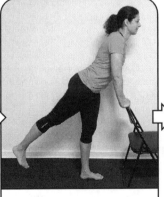

↻ **8 reps**

8. SEATED MARCH
(PAGE 68)

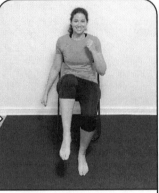

FINISH

⏱ **30 sec**

*Completing both lifts counts as one full rep.

FULL BODY TONING 1

⏱ DURATION:
4 min

🎯 GOAL:
Muscle Toning

1. LEG RAISES LEFT
(PAGE 48)

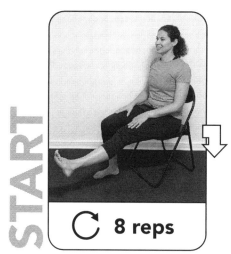

START

↻ **8 reps**

---

2. LEG RAISES RIGHT
(PAGE 48)

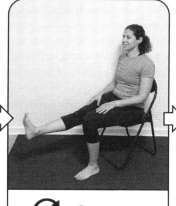

↻ **8 reps**

3. CALF RAISES
(PAGE 50)

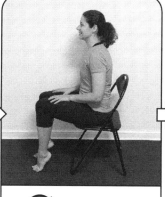

↻ **10 reps**

4. CHAIR SQUATS
(PAGE 49)

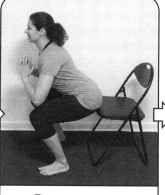

↻ **5 reps**

5. KNEE TO NOSE LEFT (PAGE 60)

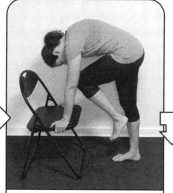

↻ **8 reps**

---

6. KNEE TO NOSE RIGHT (PAGE 60)

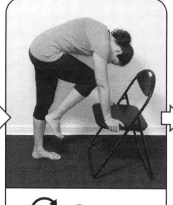

↻ **8 reps**

7. BUTTERFLY
(PAGE 80)

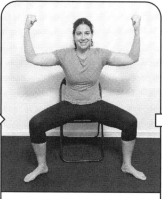

🕐 **30 sec**

8. CROSS PUNCHES
(PAGE 74)

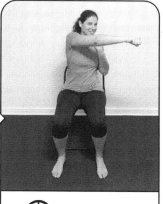

FINISH

🕐 **45 sec**

FULL BODY TONING 2

⏱ **DURATION:**
5 min

🎯 **GOAL:**
Muscle Toning

START

1. MOUNTAIN POSE OLB LEFT (PAGE 52)

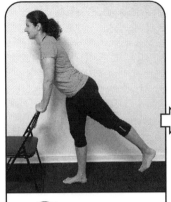

↻ **8 reps**

2. MOUNTAIN POSE OLB RIGHT (PAGE 52)

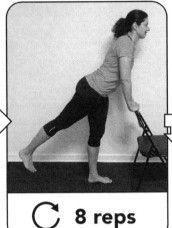

↻ **8 reps**

3. STANDING HAMSTRING CURL LEFT (P. 64)

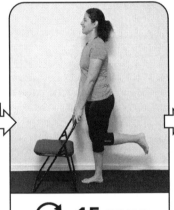

↻ **15 reps**

4. STANDING HAMSTRING CURL RIGHT (PAGE 64)

↻ **15 reps**

5. ALTERNATIVE CALF RAISES LEFT (PAGE 51)

↻ **8 reps**

6. ALTERNATIVE CALF RAISES RIGHT (PAGE 51)

↻ **8 reps**

7. STEP OUT LEFT (PAGE 54)

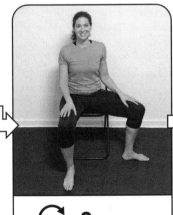

↻ **8 reps**

8. STEP OUT RIGHT (PAGE 54)

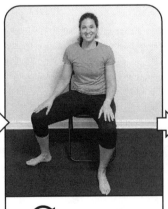

↻ **8 reps**

9. UPPERCUTS (PAGE 78)

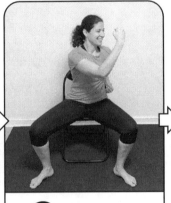

⏱ **30 sec**

10. STEP OUT AND PRESS (PAGE 82)

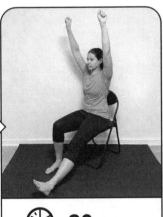

⏱ **30 sec**

FULL BODY TONING 3

DURATION:
4 min

GOAL:
Muscle Toning

1. KNEE TO NOSE LEFT (PAGE 60)

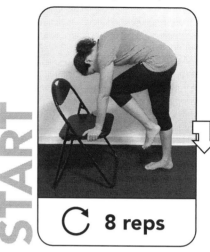

START

↻ **8 reps**

2. KNEE TO NOSE RIGHT (PAGE 60)

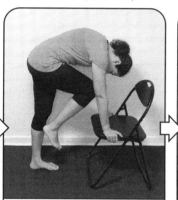

↻ **8 reps**

3. MOUNTAIN POSE OLB LEFT (PAGE 52)

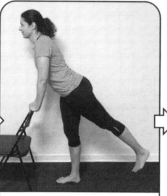

↻ **8 reps**

4. MOUNTAIN POSE OLB RIGHT (PAGE 52)

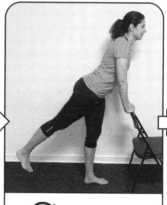

↻ **8 reps**

5. CHAIR SHUFFLE LEG (PAGE 53)

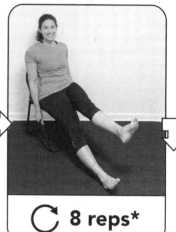

↻ **8 reps***

*Completing both lifts counts as one full rep.

6. CACTUS ARMS (PAGE 40)

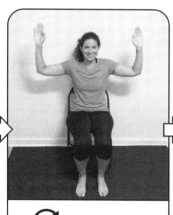

↻ **8 reps**

7. CROSS PUNCHES (PAGE 74)

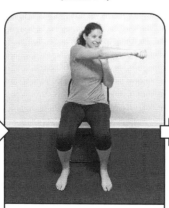

🕐 **30 sec**

8. UPPERCUTS (PAGE 78)

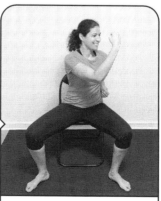

FINISH

🕐 **30 sec**

CARDIO 1

⏱ **DURATION:**

4 min

🎯 **GOAL:**

Fat Burning and Cardiovascular Health

1. SEATED KICK AND PUNCH (PAGE 66)

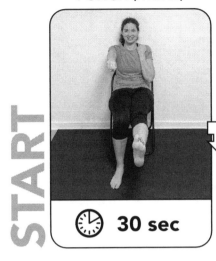

START

🕐 **30 sec**

---

2. TORSO TWIST (PAGE 70)

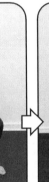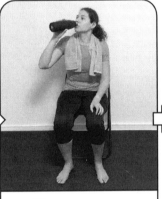

🕐 **30 sec**

3. REST

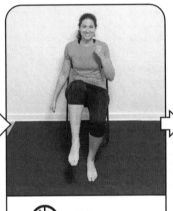

🕐 **30 sec**

4. SEATED MARCH (PAGE 68)

🕐 **30 sec**

5. STARS (PAGE 76)

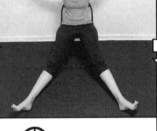

🕐 **30 sec**

---

6. REST

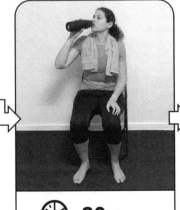

🕐 **30 sec**

7. L AND KICK (PAGE 72)

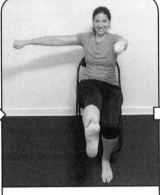

🕐 **30 sec**

8. SEATED MARCH (PAGE 68)

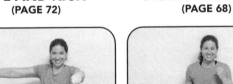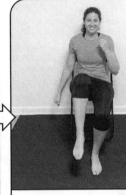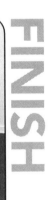

FINISH

🕐 **30 sec**

CARDIO 2

⟳ DURATION:

4 min

◎ GOAL:

Fat Burning and Cardiovascular Health

1. SEATED MARCH
(PAGE 68)

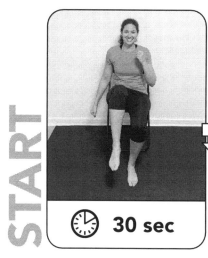

START

🕐 **30 sec**

---

2. UPPERCUTS
(PAGE 78)

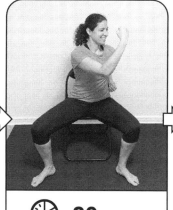

🕐 **30 sec**

3. REST

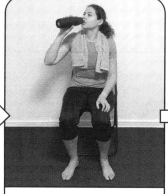

🕐 **30 sec**

4. SEATED MARCH
(PAGE 68)

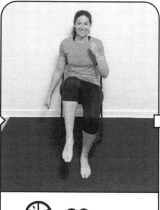

🕐 **30 sec**

5. CROSS PUNCHES
(PAGE 74)

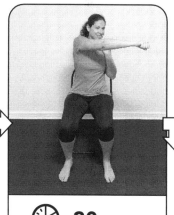

🕐 **30 sec**

---

6. REST

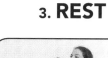

🕐 **30 sec**

7. SEATED MARCH
(PAGE 68)

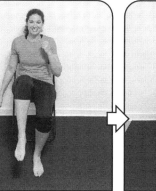

🕐 **30 sec**

8. SEATED KICK AND
PUNCH (PAGE 66)

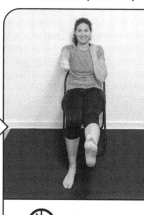
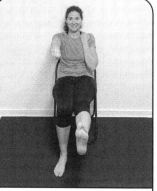

FINISH

🕐 **30 sec**

CARDIO 3

 DURATION:

4 min

GOAL:

Fat Burning and Cardiovascular Health

1. L AND KICK
(PAGE 72)

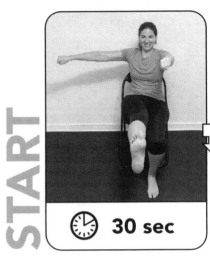

START

🕐 **30 sec**

2. STARS
(PAGE 76)

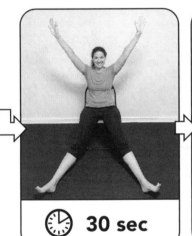

🕐 **30 sec**

3. REST

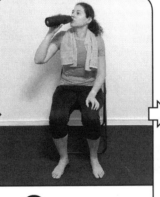

🕐 **30 sec**

4. SEATED MARCH
(PAGE 68)

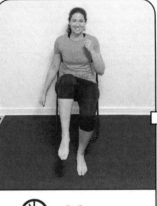

🕐 **30 sec**

5. SEATED KICK AND PUNCH (PAGE 66)

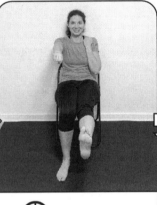

🕐 **30 sec**

6. REST

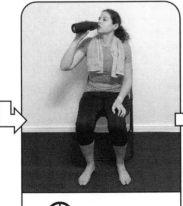

🕐 **30 sec**

7. BUTTERFLY
(PAGE 80)

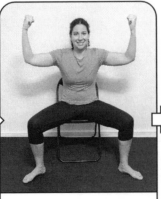

🕐 **30 sec**

8. STEP OUT AND PRESS (PAGE 82)

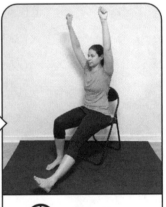

FINISH

🕐 **30 sec**

CARDIO 4

DURATION:
4 min

GOAL:
Fat Burning and
Cardiovascular Health

1. SEATED MARCH
(PAGE 68)

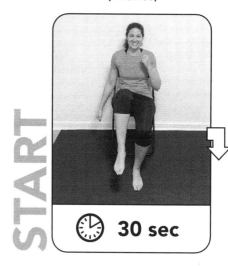

START

🕐 **30 sec**

---

2. CROSS PUNCHES
(PAGE 74)

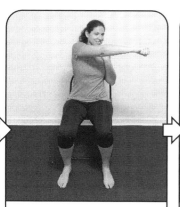

🕐 **30 sec**

3. REST

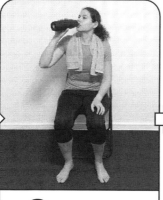

🕐 **30 sec**

4. UPPERCUTS
(PAGE 78)

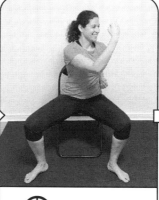

🕐 **30 sec**

5. SEATED MARCH
(PAGE 68)

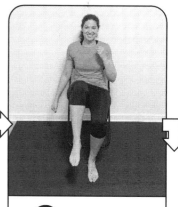

🕐 **30 sec**

---

6. REST

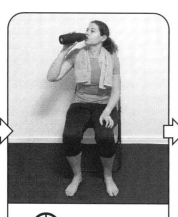

🕐 **30 sec**

7. SEATED KICK AND PUNCH (PAGE 66)

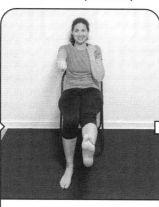

🕐 **30 sec**

8. SEATED MARCH
(PAGE 68)

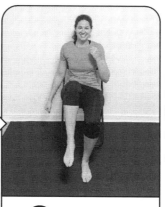

FINISH

🕐 **30 sec**

CARDIO 5

🕐 **DURATION:**

4 min

🎯 **GOAL:**

Fat Burning and Cardiovascular Health

1. STARS
(PAGE 76)

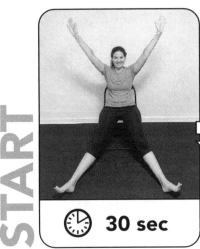

START

🕐 **30 sec**

---

2. STEP OUT AND PRESS (PAGE 82)

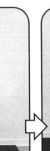
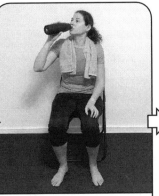

🕐 **30 sec**

3. REST

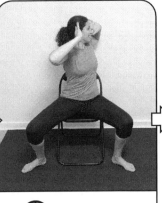

🕐 **30 sec**

4. TORSO TWIST
(PAGE 70)

🕐 **30 sec**

5. SEATED KICK AND PUNCH (PAGE 66)

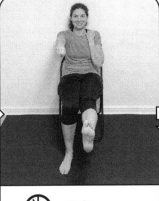

🕐 **30 sec**

---

6. REST

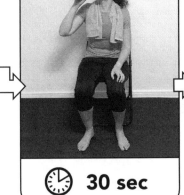

🕐 **30 sec**

7. L AND KICK
(PAGE 72)

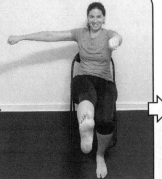

🕐 **30 sec**

8. BUTTERFLY
(PAGE 80)

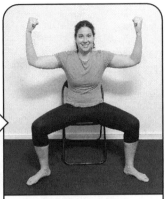

FINISH

🕐 **30 sec**

28-DAY CHALLENGE

HOW TO APPROACH THE 28-DAY CHALLENGE

Embarking on a 28-day chair yoga challenge is a commendable commitment to your well-being and fitness. As you begin this transformative journey, there are several key aspects to keep in mind to ensure you reap the maximum benefits.

Consistency is Key: The essence of any challenge lies in its regularity. To truly experience the transformative power of chair yoga, it's vital to be consistent. Dedicate a specific time each day to your practice, whether it's the early morning calm or the evening's tranquility. By making it a daily ritual, you'll not only cultivate discipline but also witness gradual improvements in your flexibility, strength, and overall well-being.

Tune In to Your Body: While consistency is crucial, it's equally important to listen to your body. Some days, you might feel energetic and ready to tackle more challenging poses, while on others, you might need something gentler. Remember, it's not about pushing your limits every day but about understanding and respecting your body's signals.

Stay Focused on Your Goals: Whether you're aiming to shed some pounds or enhance your fitness level, always keep your objectives at the forefront. When motivation wanes, remind yourself of why you started this challenge. Visualize the end result – a fitter, more agile, and healthier version of yourself. This mental image can serve as a powerful motivator on days when you need that extra push.

Visualize the Finish Line: Imagine the immense satisfaction and pride you'll feel after completing the 28 days. Visualizing this accomplishment can be a potent source of motivation. Think about the enhanced flexibility, the newfound strength, and the sense of achievement that awaits you at the end. This vision will not only keep you going but also make the journey enjoyable.

Embrace the Challenges: Like any worthwhile endeavor, there will be days when the challenge feels particularly tough. It's essential to acknowledge that these moments are a part of the journey. Instead of getting disheartened, hold yourself accountable. Remember, every time you push through a challenging day, you're one step closer to your goal. Celebrate these small victories, for they compound into significant achievements.

Remember, every workout is a step closer to becoming the best version of yourself. Keep up the great work, stay consistent, and you'll achieve your fitness goals. Believe in your strength, embrace the journey, and celebrate each small victory along the way. You've got this!

N.B.: The 28-day challenge in this book includes one warm-up and one workout for each day. Feel free to repeat the workout 1 to 3 times or more, depending on your fitness level.

28-DAY CHALLENGE

DAY 1
WARM UP:
Gentle Warm Up (P. 86)

WORKOUT*:
Full Body Toning 1 (P. 95)

DAY 2
WARM UP:
Sun Salutation (P. 85)

WORKOUT*:
Static Toning 1 (P. 90)

DAY 3
WARM UP:
Gentle Warm Up (P. 86)

WORKOUT*:
Cardio 2 (P. 99)

DAY 4
REST

DAY 5
WARM UP:
Legs Relief (P. 89)

WORKOUT*:
Legs Toning 1 (P. 92)

DAY 6
WARM UP:
Sun Salutation (P. 85)

WORKOUT*:
Cardio 4 (P. 101)

DAY 7
REST

DAY 8
WARM UP:
Gentle Warm Up (P. 86)

WORKOUT*:
Full Body Toning 2 (P. 96)

DAY 9
WARM UP:
Gentle Warm Up (P. 86)

WORKOUT*:
Static Toning 2 (P. 91)

DAY 10
WARM UP:
Sun Salutation (P. 85)

WORKOUT*:
Cardio 1 (P. 98)

DAY 11
REST

DAY 12
WARM UP:
Legs Relief (P. 89)

WORKOUT*:
Legs Toning 2 (P. 93)

DAY 13
WARM UP:
Gentle Warm Up (P. 86)

WORKOUT*:
Cardio 3 (P. 100)

DAY 14
REST

*Repeat the daily workout from 1 to 3 times, depending on your fitness level.

DAY 15

WARM UP:
Gentle Warm Up (P. 86)

WORKOUT*:
Full Body Toning 1 (P. 95)

DAY 16

WARM UP:
Gentle Warm Up (P. 86)

WORKOUT*:
Full Body Toning 3 (P. 97)

DAY 17

WARM UP:
Sun Salutation (P. 85)

WORKOUT*:
Cardio 5 (P. 102)

DAY 18

REST

DAY 19

WARM UP:
Gentle Warm Up (P. 86)

WORKOUT*:
Cardio 4 (P. 101)

DAY 20

WARM UP:
Legs Relief (P. 89)

WORKOUT*:
Legs Toning 3 (P. 94)

DAY 21

REST

DAY 22

WARM UP:
Gentle Warm Up (P. 86)

WORKOUT*:
Cardio 1 (P. 98)

DAY 23

WARM UP:
Gentle Warm Up (P. 86)

WORKOUT*:
Cardio 2 (P. 99)

DAY 24

WARM UP:
Sun Salutation (P. 85)

WORKOUT*:
Static Toning 1 (P. 90)

DAY 25

REST

DAY 26

WARM UP:
Gentle Warm Up (P. 86)

WORKOUT*:
Full Body Toning 1 (P. 95)

DAY 27

WARM UP:
Gentle Warm Up (P. 86)

WORKOUT*:
Full Body Toning 3 (P. 97)

DAY 28

REST

YOUR ACCESS CODE

cyga5465

Thank you for choosing "Chair Yoga for Weight Loss." We're excited to help you embark on your chair yoga journey!

To access our exclusive online platform, where you'll discover video tutorials for exercises, routines, and workouts designed to complement the content of this book, please follow these simple steps:

STEP 1: Using your preferred web browser and device, visit our website: **https://www.sheerfitnessvibes.com** and navigate to the 'chairyoga' section. You can access this platform on your <u>computer, tablet, or smartphone</u>.

STEP 2: In this section, a pop-up should appear, asking for an 'Access Code.' Enter the code **cyga5465** into the provided field, and the pop-up should disappear, allowing you to access the section.

STEP 3: Enjoy Your Content! Now that you have entered the code, you'll gain full access to all the chair yoga exercises, routines, and workouts corresponding to this book. Explore the platform and enjoy the benefits of chair yoga at your own pace.

> ⚠ **Important Notes:**
> If you use a different device or browser to access our website, you may need to re-enter the code.

Thank you for being a part of our chair yoga community. We're here to support you on your wellness journey, and we hope you find our platform a valuable resource to enhance your practice.

If you encounter any issues with your access code or need assistance, please don't hesitate to contact our support team at <u>support@sheerfitnessvibes.com</u>.

BONUS

As a special thank you for choosing our book, we're excited to present an exclusive bonus to complement your chair yoga routine. Introducing "Intermittent Fasting After 50" - a digital guide tailored to enhance your health and amplify the benefits of your yoga practice.

We firmly believe in the power of chair yoga as a standalone tool for weight loss and improving overall fitness. If you find fulfillment and progress through the yoga practices alone, that's wonderful! Chair yoga is a complete and effective approach in itself. However, if you're curious about amplifying your results and exploring other safe health strategies, intermittent fasting might be an intriguing addition.

Intermittent fasting isn't just a diet trend; it's a sustainable lifestyle change that has been shown to offer numerous health benefits, including improved metabolic health, increased cognitive function, and enhanced physical energy. When combined with the gentle yet effective exercises in chair yoga, intermittent fasting can be a powerful tool in managing your weight and improving overall health.

This guide provides actionable strategies and tips to safely integrate intermittent fasting into your lifestyle. Whether you're a beginner to fasting or looking to refine your approach, "Intermittent Fasting After 50" is designed to be accessible and informative for all.

To access your free digital copy of "Intermittent Fasting After 50", simply scan the QR code below or visit the URL **https://bit.ly/47usNmA**. This exclusive content is our gift to you! It's a tool to empower and guide you as you continue your wellness journey with chair yoga.

https://bit.ly/47usNmA

Made in United States
Orlando, FL
14 January 2024

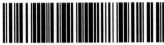